MW01254856

EVEREST
The Testing Place

EVEREST
The Testing Place

JOHN B. WEST, M.D.
Foreword by Sir Edmund Hillary

McGraw-Hill Book Company

New York • St. Louis • San Francisco • Hamburg • Mexico • Toronto

1 2 3 4 5 6 7 8 9 D O C D O C 8 7 6 5

ISBN 0-07-069502-4

LIBRARY OF CONGRESS CATALOGING IN PUBLICATION DATA

West, John Burnard.
Everest—the testing place.

Results of the American Medical Research Expedition
to Mt. Everest, 1981.
Bibliography: p.
Includes index.
1. Altitude, Influence of—Everest, Mount (China and
Nepal)   2. American Medical Research Expedition to
Mt. Everest, 1981.   3. Mountaineering—Everest, Mount
(China and Nepal)   I. American Medical Research
Expedition to Mt. Everest (1981)   II. Title.
QP82.2.A4W47   1985   612'.22'072   85-4266
ISBN 0-07-069502-4

Book design by Patrice Fodero

PREFACE

When H. W. Tilman, the eminent English explorer, was introducing his account of the 1938 Everest expedition (the fifth unsuccessful attempt) to the Royal Geographical Society in London, he remarked, "Some day, no doubt, someone will have the enviable task of adding the last chapter, in which the mountain is climbed, and writing 'Finis.' That book, we may hope, will be the last about Mount Everest."

Alas, no. There are now dozens of major books about climbing Everest, and an untold number of minor ones. So why another? My answer is that this book is different. Certainly the American Medical Research Expedition to Everest was successful in putting five people on the summit and, in the course of this, had more than its share of excitement. But the expedition was more than this. It was in part the inevitable outcome of centuries of interest in how man can survive in the oxygen-sparse atmosphere of extreme altitudes.

Ever since the Jesuit priest José deAcosta gave the first clear description of mountain sickness in the Peruvian Andes in about 1600, scientists have wondered about the effects of low oxygen on the body, and have marveled at the ability of man to adapt to this hostile environment. The dangers of low oxygen first became obvious in the late eighteenth century when the early balloonists gave dramatic accounts of blackouts and paralysis at altitudes similar to those that climbers now reach on Everest. But the human body has hidden reserves that enabled it to respond to this challenge. Men climbed higher and higher, and when the Duke of the Abruzzi reached the unheard of altitude of 7,500 meters (24,600 feet) in the Karakorum in 1909, many physiologists were forced to change their ideas on how oxygen transport occurred in the body. Consternation was even greater when E. F. Norton in 1924 on the north side of Everest got to within 300 meters (1,000 feet) of the summit without oxygen equipment. Was it possible for man to reach the highest point on earth breathing Mother Nature's air? Many scientists did their sums and thought not. The question was answered in 1978 by Reinhold Messner and Peter Habeler in their classical "oxygenless" ascent but this again only repeated the larger enigma of *how* could the body do it.

The American Medical Research Expedition to Everest was unique in that its primary objective was scientific. Sophisticated laboratories were set up at Base Camp (5,400 meters, 17,700 feet) and Camp 2 (6,300 meters, 20,700 feet), and climbers going for the summit wore physiological monitors and carried special equipment. No one had previously attempted to make measurements above 8,000 meters (26,200 feet); the expedition succeeded in getting samples of air from the lungs on the summit, and blood samples at Camp 5 (8,050 meters, 26,400 feet). These and other data were used to explain how man can not only survive, but actually do limited work at these tremendous altitudes in spite of the oxygen pressure being less than one-third of that at sea level.

We believe that this information will eventually help in the treatment of patients with severe lung and heart disease whose bodies are also oxygen starved. In addition, those readers who climb, ski, or trek at more moderate altitudes may pick up a few tips. Even the armchair explorer may derive some satisfaction from reading this account of a successful and happy expedition where climbers and scientists joined in a common purpose, and not only put another point on the scientific map, but had the experience of a lifetime doing it.

Many people have helped with this book, and it is a pleasure to acknowledge them. First, the cooperation of all members of the expedition was essential. Many have given permission for the reproduction of photographs and for the use of extensive extracts from various tapes recorded on the mountain. Special thanks are due to John Evans for contributing to the accounts of the climbing, and to Liberty Bain for her tireless and accurate secretarial assistance. The list of donors, without whom the expedition could not have taken place, is found in Appendix E.

Finally I should emphasize that this is a personal account. Although the facts are accurate, the selection reflects my interests and priorities. No doubt other members of the expedition would tell the story in a different way. I hope that this account conveys some of my exhilaration at being involved in this great adventure.

CONTENTS

CONTENTS

LIST OF
ILLUSTRATIONS

FOREWORD

by Sir Edmund Hillary

Expeditions seem to be divided into two main categories—essentially exploratory and adventurous in nature, or with an emphasis on scientific research. Each has its own place, but the scientific programs are a much less common type, and good scientific expeditions are an even more rare event.

The American Medical Research Expedition to Mt. Everest led by Dr. John West was that unique operation, a really good scientific expedition. They had their adventures in plenty, their organization and planning were of the highest order, they overcame ferocious weather conditions, and in the end they reached the summit of the mountain. But at no time did they forget their main task—to learn all they could about the physiology of human beings working hard at extreme altitudes.

The results of their research will influence the world's attitude to high-altitude acclimatization for many generations. They believe they have found answers to many of the questions that have puzzled climbers for fifty years: What exactly is acclimatization? What changes take place in the body? Why do some people function so much better at altitude than others? Can we forecast who will be good and who won't?

This book is a fascinating revelation of the complexity and remarkable adaptability of the human machine. There is only one thing we must keep in mind—in the ultimate, despite all the changes and improvements in technology, the success of a man on a high mountain is the attitude of the man himself—his energy, his motivation, his enthusiasm.

Dr. John West's party had all of these qualities plus a complete dedication to science. They made a formidable and effective team, and their scientific results will have justified all the support and help they received.

Sir Edmund Hillary

EVEREST
The Testing Place

1
SCENARIO

Not just "because it is there"[1]

October 24, 1981. Strange events occur at the summit of Mt. Everest, a place that has seen more than its share of human drama. At about noon two climbers appear on the narrow southeast ridge, and carefully pick their way up. They lean into the fierce jet-stream wind that rips over the highest peak in the world. With their oxygen masks and extravagant clothing they look like something out of *Star Wars* on some remote planet. However, they are not the first to go this way in the last few days, as can be seen from the footprints that they meticulously follow, stepping into each one to lessen the chance of slipping and falling 8,000 feet into Nepal on one side of the ridge, or even further into Tibet on the other. We can sense the mixture of elation, relief, and exhaustion that they feel when they finally stand on the summit, the final point of years of planning. So far so good.

One of the climbers rummages around in his backpack and brings out a box to measure barometric pressure and temperature. He makes careful readings and then records the information on a small tape recorder that he pulls out of a pocket of his pile jacket. When this is replayed later the sounds of his breathless voice are almost drowned by the roar of the wind like a passing express train. Next he brings out a metal contraption that looks like some

1

extraplanetary musical instrument. He loads this with a cartridge of sampling tubes, and proceeds to make a series of rapid exhalations into it. By these maneuvers he captures for later analysis samples of air that come from deep inside his lung. All this time a small tape recorder is running in a pocket of a special vest that he is wearing next to his skin where his body warmth keeps it from freezing. Later this tape will be played back to give his electrocardiogram and other signals.

The astute observer might be able to detect a difference in attitude between the climber who is carrying out these measurements, and his sherpa companion who is anxious to get down before the piercing wind starts to numb his fingers and toes. But Dr. Chris Pizzo is not to be hurried. "Got to do science" he says. "Very important." Sherpa Young Tenzing is understandably confused by this behavior, as he and the other sherpas have been all along on this odd expedition. "We have reached the top, what more do you want?" he seems to say.

Pizzo now indulges in some relaxation.[2] He tosses a Frisbee downwind into Tibet. Being made of plastic it would probably last for many months under ordinary conditions. Up here where the below-zero temperatures slow down decomposition to an imperceptible rate it will be preserved for years as a monument to Pizzo's idiosyncrasy. "Someone's going to have to use artificial means to break my Frisbee record," he observes later. Now some photographs, and at last it is time to go down.

The two climbers carefully descend the narrow ridge very much aware that many before them have come to grief by losing concentration on a descent after the exhilaration of reaching a tough summit. One slip can mean a fall of thousands of feet into the Western Cwm of Nepal on their right, or down the steep Kangshung face of Tibet on their left. Again they follow the bootmarks left by Chris Kopczynski and Sherpa Sungdare who reached the summit three days previously. Pizzo and Young Tenzing glance down to the right and see Camp 2 way below. It is 8,000 feet down, and the tents appear as tiny dots. If they look carefully they can just make out a slightly larger dot that is the structure housing the highest laboratory in the world.

This laboratory has been the scene of intense activity every day and far into most nights for the last three weeks. While the gasoline generators, assisted by a bank of solar panels, have been chugging away charging the batteries, scientists and climbers have been pedaling to exhaustion on a stationary bicycle. An electronic gadget clamped to the subject's ear records the level of oxygen in the blood, and astonishing low values have been obtained. Studies made during sleep have shown striking unevenness of breathing—most climbers stop breathing altogether for some seconds and the oxygen in the blood

2

plummets. Dozens of blood samples have been taken; some have been analyzed in the laboratory while many others have been frozen for transport back to the U.S. In other tests the subject has tried to remember strings of words or draw patterns to determine whether the low oxygen has affected his brain.

At Base Camp another 3,000 feet below, but still nearly 18,000 feet high, more experiments are being done in a similar laboratory. In addition to the measurements on the climbers and scientists, some sherpas are also riding the bicycle and breathing into various bags. We are all aware that the sherpas can tolerate these altitudes very much better than we can, and we want to know why. Some, particularly the younger sherpas, cooperate readily, but the older ones look at the blood-drawing syringes suspiciously.

Back at the summit there is more activity, and very nearly tragedy. Some three hours after Pizzo and Young Tenzing have left, another figure appears climbing alone. He is moving slowly and cautiously because he knows that with no rope holding him any false step is likely to be his last. Only a handful of people have climbed Everest solo, and fewer still have survived. Dr. Peter Hackett finally reaches the top, but by now it is nearly 4 o'clock in the afternoon, too late to reach his tent 2,600 feet below before dark. If the tape recorder running in his vest pocket shows a surprisingly high heart rate it may be because he is increasingly apprehensive about getting off this mountain alive.

After a few hurried photographs on the summit he starts down. The narrow ridge is tricky. About 200 feet below the summit he arrives at the Hillary Step, one of the most difficult obstacles on the whole route. In fact, it was partly because of this steep section that Hackett decided to give up on a summit attempt in the morning after his sherpa partner became too cold to continue. Only after he was reassured by Chris Pizzo that secure steps were in place around this treacherous pitch did he decide to try a solo attempt.

Hackett gingerly begins to climb down in a crack between two rocks. It is difficult to see where to put his next step because his oxygen mask obscures his view as he looks down. Suddenly he realizes that the snow is too soft to bear his weight, and a moment later he is falling headlong and unroped toward the valley 8,000 feet below. Miraculously one boot snags on a protruding rock after he has fallen 10 or 15 feet, and he finds himself suspended upside down, over 28,000 feet high on Mt. Everest, with no one to help, and the evening approaching. At first he panics and rips off his oxygen mask but this only increases his breathlessness. His goggles hurtle down somewhere into the valley below. He probes with his ice axe until he finds a solid point, and then gradually rights himself. Astonishingly he finds a rope fixed to the rock, presumably left behind by some unknown previous expedition, and he grabs it. Severely shaken, he makes another step down only to fall another 10 feet as the snow gives way

3

again. Finally he recovers his composure enough to continue down to Pizzo who has been waiting for him 1,000 feet below. They descend together in the dark to their tent at Camp 5, which they reach at 8 o'clock. They are both safe now but Hackett has more than once today been within a hair's breadth of death.

How do two physicians find themselves on the summit of the world's highest mountain? Why are two tons of scientific equipment carried in for a month on the backs of porters and yaks, and then hauled up to an altitude of 21,000 feet to make the world's highest laboratory? This book tells the story of the expedition, including why it was put together and what was learned. Together with the exhilaration of success and the agony of failure there is the underlying purpose of a serious and unique scientific experiment.

When George Mallory, the notable Everest pioneer, was asked why climb Everest, he gave the well-known enigmatic reply, "Because it is there." Indeed, Mallory was eloquent on the absence of material gain from attempting to climb the mountain. "The first question which you will ask and which I must try to answer is this, 'What is the use of climbing Mount Everest?' and my answer must at once be, 'It is no use.' There is not the slightest prospect of any gain whatsoever. Oh, we may learn a little about the behaviour of the human body at high altitudes, where there is only a third of an atmosphere, and possibly medical men may turn our observation to some account for the purposes of aviation. But otherwise nothing will come of it. We shall not bring back a single bit of gold or silver, not a gem, nor any coal or iron. We shall not find a foot of earth that can be planted with crops to raise food. It's no use.

"So, if you cannot understand that there is something in man which responds to the challenge of this mountain and goes to meet it, that the struggle is the struggle of life itself upward and forever upward, then you won't see why we go. What we get from this adventure is just sheer joy. And joy is, after all, the end of life. We do not live to eat and make money. We eat and make money to be able to enjoy life. That is what life means and what life is for."[3]

Perhaps our expedition had the distinction of being the first to attempt Everest primarily for other reasons. As Dr. Lahiri, the chief Base Camp scientist, quipped, "Not because it's there, but because of the air!" In fact the thinness of the air is the basis of the body's problems at high altitude, as we shall see in the next chapter.

2

BACKGROUND

---

*"The aire . . .
so subtile and delicate"*[1]

Why lug two tons of laboratory equipment up to an altitude of 6,300 meters (20,700 feet) to study man at high altitude? Basically there are two reasons. The first is practical; we hope to derive information that will ultimately be useful in treating patients with serious lung and heart disease. The second is purely scientific; we want to know more about how man can tolerate severe oxygen deprivation.

As a climber goes higher and higher, the amount of oxygen in the air decreases because the air pressure steadily falls. At the summit of Mt. Everest the air pressure is about one-third of its sea-level value, and as a result of this the amount of oxygen available to the climber's lungs is reduced. Consequently, when he is near the summit of Mt. Everest he has extremely low levels of oxygen in his blood. This is by far the most severe oxygen deprivation that normal man ever encounters. Climbing Mt. Everest without supplementary oxygen is therefore the greatest respiratory challenge that exists.

Now, some patients with chronic bronchitis or emphysema find themselves in a similar predicament. In this instance it is not the lack of oxygen in the air that is to blame, but rather the fact that their diseased lungs are inefficient at transferring the oxygen from the air into the blood. But irrespective of the

5

reason, these patients also have greatly reduced amounts of oxygen in their blood. By studying climbers under these exceptional conditions we hope to learn more about how the body can respond to disease.

A note of caution should be sounded about how quickly we can expect the findings from this type of research to be translated into changes in the way we treat patients. It would be very satisfying, of course, if we could point to some therapeutic advance that came about as a direct result of our expedition. Indeed, newspaper reporters often ask very direct questions on this point. For example, every expedition member has heard the question—"tell me how the results of your research at high altitude help the average patient with severe lung disease."

If only medical research were as easy as this! But the way modern research progresses is that we choose an important, poorly understood area (such as the effects of severe oxygen deprivation on the body), and do careful measurements in a situation that is likely to provide new information. The underlying belief is that such work, together with other related studies, will ultimately lead to a better understanding of disease, and thus to improvements in treatment. It is this basic credo that keeps many people fossicking away on some problem in medical research even though nothing new turns up for long periods of time.

The second reason for studying people under these extreme conditions is the intrinsic scientific question of how the body adapts to oxygen deprivation. Man has a remarkable ability to do this. For example, consider the reduced atmospheric pressure at the summit of Mt. Everest. A normal person exposed to this deprivation in a low-pressure chamber would lose consciousness within a minute or so. By contrast, the acclimatized climber not only remains conscious without supplementary oxygen but can at the same time perform the considerable work of climbing to the summit.

This ability of the body to continue to function in the face of a dramatic reduction of oxygen in the air comes about through a series of changes that physicians call "acclimatization." Acclimatization to high altitude is one of the best examples in the whole of physiology of how the body changes to cope with a hostile environment. The changes that occur include an increase in both the rate and depth of breathing, an increase in the number of oxygen-carrying red cells in the blood, and other less obvious adaptations. We shall meet this subject again and again because our expedition's scientific program was focused on the success or otherwise of the body's acclimatization to high altitude.

The story of man's developing understanding of the effects of high altitude on the human body is colorful. Anyone who goes to a high altitude is aware of the combination of headache, fatigue, loss of appetite, and insomnia that

6

is called "mountain sickness." One of the earliest accounts of mountain sickness was given by the Jesuit missionary José deAcosta, who accompanied the early Spanish conquistadores of Peru in the sixteenth century. He described how as he traveled over a high mountain, "I was suddenly surprised with so mortall and strange a pang, that I was ready to fall from the top to the ground." He went on: "I was surprised with such pangs of straining and casting, as I thought to cast out my heart too—for having cast up meate, fleugme, and choller, both yellow and greene; in the end I cast up blood with the straining of my stomacke. . . . I therefore perswade myself, that the element of the aire is there so subtile and delicate, as it is not proportionable with the breathing of man, which requires a more grosse and temperate aire."[2] The last was a remarkably perceptive statement considering that it was not yet known that air had weight. This discovery had to wait for Evangelista Torricelli almost 50 years later.

Actually, the Chinese were aware of the deleterious effects of high altitude long before this. *The Tseen Han Shoo*, which dates from about 30 B.C. during the Han Dynasty, describes the route from the Western Regions to the Hindu Kush (in modern Afghanistan): it crosses "the Great Headache Mountain, the Little Headache Mountain . . . men's bodies become feverish, they lose color, and are attacked with headache and vomiting; the asses and cattle being all in like condition."[3]

Some of the early theories of the cause of mountain sickness seem quaint today. One popular notion was that the low air pressure caused weakening of the joint between the hip bone and the pelvis. It was argued that the pressure of the air was important in pressing the two together, and that at high altitude loss of this force required the hip muscles to work harder, and thus become fatigued. Needless to say, this makes no sense because all the pressures within the body decrease along with the outside pressure.

An even more elaborate explanation was given by a Dr. Cunningham who believed that atmospheric electricity was the culprit. The good doctor came up with a devious explanation based on the role of electricity attracting blood to the head in the northern hemisphere, and to the lower parts of the body in the southern hemisphere. He believed that mountain sickness caused apoplexy in Europe but resulted in fainting in the South American Andes! Yet another theory was that distension of air in the abdomen as a result of the low atmospheric pressure interfered with breathing and circulation. Actually we now know (chiefly as a result of the work of the great French physiologist Paul Bert) that the reduction of air pressure by itself has no effect on the body. The important factor is the decrease in the amount of oxygen.

Some of the most dramatic observations of the effects of low oxygen on the body were made by the early balloonists. These intrepid explorers had a large impact on the development of knowledge of the physiologic effects of high altitude, especially of rapid severe oxygen deprivation. Until the Montgolfier brothers astounded the citizens of Paris with the first manned hot-air balloon flight in November 1783, the only other way to expose man to low pressures was by mountain climbing. However, climbing involved so much exertion that many physiologists attributed the deleterious effects of high altitude to fatigue, as we have seen.

One of the most colorful accounts of the physical and mental effects of low oxygen was a balloon ascent by Glaisher and Coxwell in 1862. James Glaisher was the chief meteorologist at the Royal Observatory in Greenwich, and he became interested in the possibility of making observations from balloons. After several attempts to delegate this responsibility to younger men, he made the ascents himself at the age of 53. Henry Coxwell, a dentist who had become a professional balloonist, was in charge of the balloon, and the two made a series of scientific flights. In one, the balloon rapidly rose to an altitude estimated at 7 miles (over 11,000 meters, or 36,000 feet), considerably higher than the summit of Mt. Everest. High in their flight Glaisher collapsed, and Coxwell tried to vent hydrogen from the balloon, but because his hands were paralyzed by the low oxygen, he had to seize the cord with his teeth, and dip his head two or three times! Just as remarkable was the fact that when the balloon eventually landed, Glaisher felt "no inconvenience," and walked over 7 miles to the nearest village because they came down in a remote country area.[4]

However, the most famous of balloon ascents in this period was that undertaken in the balloon "Zenith" in 1875 by the three French balloonists, Tissandier, Croce-Spinelli, and Sivel. Their balloon reached an altitude estimated to be 8,600 meters (28,000 feet), and when it returned to the ground Croce-Spinelli and Sivel had succumbed to the oxygen lack. Tragically, although oxygen had been provided for the aeronauts, there was not enough, and furthermore it was difficult to inhale because it was bubbled through bottles of water to remove an unpleasant odor. The disaster caused a sensation in France. It might be added that there was a good deal of competitive ballooning at this time with each balloonist trying to outdo the other with little notion of the hazards of extreme altitudes. For example, in the funeral oration that followed the "Zenith" tragedy, Pastor Coquerel remarked that, "they say that an Englishman could live and make observations above 8,000 meters: the flag we carry must float higher yet!" Sad to say, such jingoism is not unknown in modern mountaineering.

More serious investigations into the bodily changes that occur at high altitude began toward the end of the nineteenth century. A key figure in high-altitude physiology at that time was Paul Bert, a French physiologist who worked in Paris in the 1860s and 1870s. Bert was the first to prove that the deleterious effects of high altitude were caused by the low pressure of oxygen.[5] He exposed animals to air in low-pressure chambers, and compared their responses to animals exposed to low-oxygen concentrations at normal sea-level pressures. By doing this he was able to demonstrate convincingly that the partial pressure of oxygen was the important factor.[6]

Although Bert's experiments were extensive, not everybody was convinced by his findings. One who was not was the Italian physiologist Angelo Mosso, who built the first high-altitude station for physiological research in the 1890s. Mosso persuaded Queen Margherita of Italy, an ardent mountaineer herself, to provide funds for the building, and it was placed at an altitude of 4,570 meters (15,000 feet) on one of the peaks of Monta Rosa in the Italian Alps. Several important observations were made there including the unevenness of breathing during sleep, which is common at high altitude and which we studied in our Camp 2 and Base Camp laboratories. However, the station was rather inaccessible, and the notable English physiologist Joseph Barcroft thought the conditions "too rigorous"; he remarked that "the difficulty of transport greatly restricts the possibilities both of research and gastronomy."

A series of research expeditions to high altitude during this century made great contributions to our understanding of high-altitude medicine and physiology. One of the earliest expeditions was in 1911 when an international group went to the summit of Pike's Peak near Colorado Springs. The four scientists were two Englishmen, C. G. Douglas and J. S. Haldane, and two Americans, Yandell Henderson and Edward Schneider. The summit observatory that was used as a laboratory is at an altitude of 4,300 meters (14,110 feet), and has the advantage of easy accessibility. At this time there was a great dispute going on in the physiological world about how oxygen was transferred by the lungs into the blood. One group championed by Haldane argued that the lungs actively secreted the oxygen so that the resulting pressure of oxygen in the blood could be higher than that in the air of the lungs. This "vitalist" view of the lungs would make them analogous to the body's endocrine glands that actively secrete various substances. The opposing view was that the lung was a purely passive organ, and that oxygen simply diffused across the barrier between the air and the blood, from an area of high pressure to one of low pressure. Subsequent research has borne out the latter view. However, on this expedition Haldane and his co-workers believed they obtained very strong evidence of oxygen secretion, and the results influenced the progress of physiology for many years.[7]

Partly in response to this, another international expedition was organized in the winter of 1921–1922, this time to Cerro de Pasco at an altitude of 4,330 meters (14,200 feet) in the Peruvian Andes. The leader was Joseph Barcroft. The hypothesis of oxygen secretion was carefully tested but no evidence for it was found. Many other important studies were made, including the rate of increase of red blood cells that occurs as a result of acclimatization, and changes in the relationship between oxygen pressure and concentration in the blood.[8]

One of the most significant outcomes of this expedition was the interest that it aroused in the physiology of permanent residents of high altitudes. The Peruvian and Chilean Andes contain the highest towns and villages in the world, and they have become important sites for the study of the effects of high altitude. The expedition party was enormously impressed by the capacity of the residents for physical work, and they were astonished at the popularity of energetic sports such as football (soccer). Nevertheless, Barcroft concluded that "all dwellers at high altitudes [are] persons of impaired physical and mental powers," a sentiment that incensed the Peruvian physician Carlos Monge. He and his pupil, Alberto Hurtado, subsequently embarked on an extensive study of these permanent residents. It could be argued that the development of this influential Peruvian school of high-altitude physiology dated from Barcroft's expedition, and possibly from this unguarded remark.

Monge vigorously defended the natives of the Peruvian Andes. He even asserted that Barcroft's conclusions were formed when he was unknowingly suffering from mountain sickness, and thus by implication could hardly be held responsible for them! In Barcroft's defense it should be pointed out that this notion of the inferior performance of the inhabitants of Cerro de Pasco was only briefly referred to in his book, while the emphasis was on their remarkably high working capacity.

However, stimulated in part by Barcroft's remarks, Monge and Hurtado went on to analyze how these high-altitude dwellers have adapted to the "climatic aggression" (as they called it) of high altitude. They pointed out that one of the major differences between the Spanish conquistadores and the resident native population in the sixteenth and seventeenth centuries was that the Spanish could reproduce only by going to low altitudes. Monge also unearthed some interesting facts about the Incas who had developed their sophisticated civilization in the high Andes centuries before. He noted, for example, that the Incas recognized the advantages of high-altitude acclimatization to such an extent that they kept two armies; one operated only at high altitudes while the other fought only on the lower plains.[9]

Another important international high-altitude expedition took place in 1935 under the scientific leadership of Dr. D. B. Dill.[10] This remarkable scientist is now in his 90s but he remains actively interested in high-altitude physiology.

We were delighted when he agreed to serve as one of the scientific advisers to our expedition. The 1935 expedition chose to go to Aucanquilcha in the Chilean Andes because of a sulfur mine there at an altitude of 5,800 meters (19,000 feet), although the miners live about 450 meters (1,500 feet) below this. Attempts have been made to persuade the workers to live at the mine but these have always failed. The miners' camp at 5,350 meters (17,500 feet) is probably the highest permanent population in the world.

During this expedition some members climbed to the top of Aucanquilcha Mountain, altitude 6,100 meters (20,000 feet), where they set up a temporary camp for simple measurements. One impressive feat was the taking of an arterial blood sample of a member of the expedition while he lay on the frozen ground. This was the highest arterial blood sample ever taken until our expedition broke the record 46 years later. Blood from an artery is more difficult to collect than blood from a vein, and there is more risk from possible clotting difficulties. The main emphasis of this expedition was on blood chemistry, that is, the changes in the various constituents of the blood as a result of high altitude. Indeed, the results formed the basis of our current knowledge on the subject.

A particularly important expedition from our point of view took place in 1960–61. This was the Himalayan Scientific and Mountaineering Expedition led by Sir Edmund Hillary, with Dr. L. G. C. E. Pugh as scientific director.[11] The design of the expedition was complex but ingenious, with the program spread over nine months between September 1960 and May 1961. In September two groups trekked into the Everest region from Kathmandu. One took along a prefabricated hut, which they erected on a glacier at an altitude of 5,800 meters (19,000 feet) just southeast of the lovely mountain, Ama Dablam. This site was chosen because of its relatively easy accessibility, and its safety for such a high altitude. The second group trekked into the Rowaling area ostensibly to search for the Yeti or abominable snowman. In addition to this exotic objective the party carried out studies on the wildlife of this little-known region. Included in this group was Marlin Perkins, ex-director of the St. Louis Zoo, and well known to millions of television viewers through his popular program "Wild Kingdom."

The second part of the expedition took place at the end of the fall when the hut was occupied by a group of physiologists who spent the winter studying their gradual acclimatization to this great altitude. The design of the hut proved to be very effective, and it greatly influenced the subsequent design of the laboratory that we used at Base Camp (5,400 meters, 17,700 feet) on the present expedition. The building, which became known as the Silver Hut because of its aluminum paint coating, was constructed of curved panels con-

11

sisting of 3 inches of foam plastic sandwiched between marine plywood sheets. The structure was 22 feet long by 10 feet wide, and the panels were doweled so that the whole structure could be assembled in one day.

Wintering in this remote, high region was surprisingly comfortable. One end of the hut served as a laboratory, and was provided with electrical light and power from a gasoline generator and wind-driven dynamo. In the center of the hut was a large paraffin stove that served as a cooking area and heater. Eight bunks were set up in the other end, and the hut was continuously occupied by six to eight physiologists from December 1960 until April 1961.

During the winter they carried out an elaborate program of research. This centered on the responses of the heart and lungs to exercise, but additional investigations studied the control of breathing, the changes that occur in the blood, and the reasons for the relentless loss of weight experienced by everybody. Not all was work, however. In the late afternoons the scientists often skied on the glacier. However, the skiers paid dearly for a five-minute downhill schuss: it was followed by half an hour's breathless walk back up the mountain while they carried their skis.

In the spring the expedition moved to Mount Makalu (8,475 meters [27,790 feet]), the world's fifth highest mountain. This had been climbed previously by a French expedition in 1955, but Hillary's plan was to attempt the mountain without supplementary oxygen. If this had been successful it would have been the highest "oxygenless" summit at that time. A new mountaineering group joined them in the spring, and one of the interesting questions was how the performance of the party who had spent the entire winter in the hut would compare with that of newcomers who had only the usual two-month acclimatization. In the event there was very little difference between the two groups during the climb on Makalu. In fact, it was suggested that the long wintering period had sapped some of that group's vitality, and there is little doubt that this altitude of 5,800 meters (19,000 feet) is not only too high for permanent habitation but also too high for optimal acclimatization.

In addition to the main scientific program of the expedition, a stationary bicycle was carried up to the Makalu Col (7,440 meters [24,400 feet]), and measurements of maximal work capacity and oxygen consumption were made on two of the doctors. These remain the highest direct measurements of work capacity ever made. The maximal oxygen consumption was down to about a third of what it is at sea level. As a joke I used to state on my curriculum vitae (résumé) that I hold the world's record for measured oxygen consumption for 7,440 meters (24,400 feet). However, this was measured on only two people, and one subject, Dr. Michael Ward, probably had some lung disease at the time so the record is really by default!

The expedition did not succeed in reaching the summit of Makalu. Temperatures were very cold, and the winds were exceptionally fierce. One of the assault team, Peter Mulgrew from New Zealand, suddenly collapsed about 120 meters (400 feet) from the summit, apparently because of a blood clot in his lungs. The ensuing ten days were a nightmare as we tried to get Mulgrew off the mountain alive. He subsequently lost both legs below the knees because of severe frostbite, and developed an addiction to the pain-killing drugs, but gallantly fought back to become a successful businessman in Auckland and a competitive yachtsman. He was killed recently in a tragic crash of a commercial airline scenic flight to Antarctica where he was narrating the sights.

The Himalayan Scientific and Mountaineering Expedition was an outstanding success from the scientific point of view. It remains the most extensive study of the responses of normal man to an altitude of 5,800 meters (19,000 feet), and the design of the expedition by Hillary and Pugh was a brilliant fusion of the scientific and the climbing objectives. It had a great influence on the planning of our expedition. Not only was the laboratory that we used at Base Camp very much based on the design of the Silver Hut, but three members of the previous expedition, Jim Milledge, Sukhamay Lahiri, and myself, took part in the present expedition. Added to this, Hillary agreed to lend his name to our expedition as Expedition Advisor so that it can reasonably be argued that AMREE was the son of HSME.

There have been other expeditions with medical research objectives since the Himalayan Scientific and Mountaineering Expedition, but none as ambitious. One of unusual interest was the Italian expedition to Mt. Everest in 1973 during which a sophisticated laboratory was set up at Base Camp at an altitude of 5,400 meters (17,600 feet), and an extensive series of measurements was made on climbers who had been above 8,000 meters (26,000 feet). This expedition was remarkable for the outstanding logistic support provided by the Italian army. Two helicopters helped to lift supplies into the Western Cwm at an altitude of over 6,000 meters (20,000 feet). One of the helicopters crashed there (fortunately there were no injuries), and it is said that a piece of it recently emerged at the bottom of the icefall. The Khumbu icefall between the Western Cwm and Base Camp is continually moving, though very slowly, and it occasionally spits out grim reminders of earlier expeditions.

Another notable high-altitude research program was carried out for several years on a 5,300 meter (17,500 foot) high plateau near Mt. Logan in the Canadian Yukon. Organized by Dr. Charles Houston, a veteran mountaineer with a lifelong interest in high-altitude medicine, this program operated for several years every summer, chiefly studying the acclimatization processes in normal subjects flown to this remote area. Our own expedition received enormous support from Charlie Houston. He was one of our scientific advisers and also led one of the treks to the Base Camp for friends of the expedition. When you meet him and see his youthful appearance it is difficult to believe that he led the first successful ascent of Nanda Devi (7,821 meters [25,660 feet]) in 1936.

So far we have considered high-altitude experiments carried out in the natural laboratory of a mountain. But it is also possible to expose people to low pressures for extended periods of time in a low-pressure chamber. Such chambers are employed extensively for studies of acute oxygen deprivation, for example by the air forces. However, their use in studying long-term acclimatization involves many logistical problems. To tolerate the very low oxygen pressure that exists near the summit of Mt. Everest, the minimum period of acclimatization is around six to eight weeks. It is no small matter to confine a group of people for this length of time, and there are very few facilities that will allow this. Moreover, the psychological effects of being cooped up for such a long period are considerable. For example, it has not yet been determined whether individuals who spend such a long period in a low-pressure chamber can remain fit and accomplish the high exercise levels that are seen on research expeditions to high altitudes.

Nevertheless, one successful low-pressure-chamber study has been completed, the so-called "Operation Everest." This was conducted at the U.S. Naval Air Station in Pensacola, Florida, in 1946 by Drs. Charles Houston and Richard Riley.[12] Four naval recruits were exposed to successively lower pressures in a 10 x 12 x 7 foot chamber over a period of 32 days. The barometric pressure was gradually reduced from the sea level value of 760 millimeters of mercury to about 320, and there were two short "excursions" to much lower pressures corresponding to the summit of Mt. Everest. Useful information on the transport of oxygen in the body was obtained, although unfortunately no attempt was made to study maximal exercise, so it is difficult to know how well acclimatized the subjects were at the end of the experiment. As I write this, "Operation Everest II" is being planned to take place in a U.S. Army facility, and there is no doubt that if the logistical problems can be overcome, a low-pressure chamber will make it much easier to carry out some valuable experiments on high-altitude physiology, especially those associated with appreciable risk. Naturally it is much easier to transfer a subject to a hospital from a facility like this than from a remote mountain top.

These expeditions and research programs have helped immensely our understanding of how high altitude affects man. In addition, several exceptional climbs to high altitudes have had an impact on physiologists' thinking. For example, when the Duke of the Abruzzi reached the extraordinary altitude of

7,500 meters (24,600 feet) on Chogolisa in the Karakorum Mountains in 1909 without supplementary oxygen, physiologists were dumbfounded because many had previously believed that it was impossible for man to survive in such an oxygen-deprived environment. Indeed, Douglas and Haldane made some calculations of the oxygen pressures in the lungs and blood of the redoubtable Duke and concluded that his lungs must have actively secreted oxygen into the blood to enable him to accomplish what he did.

Similar astonishment greeted the climb by Norton and Sommervell to over 8,530 meters (28,000 feet) on the north side of Everest in the famous expedition of 1924. These climbers were not using oxygen equipment, and Norton's account vividly describes the excruciatingly slow going at this altitude. It took him an hour to gain 30 vertical meters (100 feet), though he stuck to his opinion that it would be possible for a fresh and fit party to reach the top of Everest without oxygen. This was the expedition on which Mallory and Irvine mysteriously disappeared; they were last seen climbing toward the summit at an altitude of 8,400 meters (27,500 feet), and to this day there are arguments about whether they were successful or not.

The most dramatic ascent of all was by Messner and Habeler in May 1978. They did indeed reach the summit of Everest, 8,848 meters (29,028 feet) high, without supplementary oxygen. Both their accounts emphasized how close they were to the limit of human endurance in this rarified atmosphere. Messner wrote of collapsing on the snow every 10 or 15 steps on the final summit ridge, and when he eventually got to the top he recalled, "in my state of spiritual abstraction, I no longer belong to myself and to my eyesight. I am nothing more than a single, narrow, gasping lung, floating over the mists and the summits." This remarkable ascent stimulated several physiologists to rethink the mechanisms of oxygen transfer from the air to the tissues under these exceptional conditions. We did the same, and the results helped us to identify what measurements would be particularly valuable on our forthcoming expedition.[13]

So this was the background against which we decided to mount an expedition to obtain measurements on how man is able to function successfully at these extreme altitudes. As is so often the case, the actual design of the expedition developed gradually over a number of years. The earliest recollection I have was a meeting with Jim Milledge in London in September 1974. I was on sabbatical leave at the time, finishing a book, and of course Jim was an old friend from the 1960 expedition. He had kept up his interest in high-altitude medicine, and had carried out two or three small research projects while hill walking in Wales or skiing in Switzerland. We talked about the possibilities of going back to the Himalaya, and making some simple measurements of lung and heart function. Plans included breathing rate and volume, obtaining electrocardiograms, measuring the oxygen content of the blood using a device (oximeter) on the ear, samples of air from the depths of the lungs, further studies of red-cell concentration and acidity of the blood, and absorption of food by the gut. All these measurements were subsequently done on our expedition. We also discussed some more ambitious projects, such as putting a catheter into the heart to measure the pressure on the right side, and taking small pieces of leg muscle from some subjects using special needles. Both of these projects would be of considerable scientific importance, but they were abandoned as being too uncomfortable or too dangerous, or both.

At this time we were considering a small group of perhaps three or four scientists who would accompany a regular climbing expedition. Recently Arnold Heine, a New Zealander, had written to Jim about taking part in a New Zealand expedition to Everest planned for 1977. We began to seriously consider the possibility of attaching a small scientific group to this expedition, and in early 1976 I applied for a research contract to the National Heart, Lung and Blood Institute in Bethesda, Maryland, to carry out a program of measurements above 7,500 meters (25,000 feet). This institute is one of the dozen or so U.S. National Institutes of Health that fund a large portion of man-related life science research in the United States. The measurements were to include breathing rate and volume, electrocardiogram, samples of air from the depths of the lungs, and oxygen consumption. One idea was to telemeter data from climbers near the summit of Everest down to Camp 1 just above the Khumbu icefall. At this time there was no thought of setting up a laboratory hut above the icefall or putting a special scientific tent on the South Col.

This contract was funded largely through the strong support of Dr. Claude Lenfant, then director of the Lung Division of the institute, and we started to look into measuring equipment. One important find was a miniature slow-running tape recorder that could record four channels of data over twenty-four hours, and which was small enough to be carried by a climber. Various tests on this recorder, which had the trade name "Medilog," were made during the spring of 1976.

It gradually became clear that linking up with the 1977 New Zealand expedition to Everest was just not going to work. They were very short of money, and they certainly could not afford the luxury of a scientific addition, even though we had guaranteed to look after our own expenses. But at about this time a small team of Americans was setting out to attempt to climb Everest in the fall of 1976. This expedition had had severe financial problems but was saved by the Columbia Broadcasting System who offered to cover the costs of the expedition in return for being allowed to make a television film of it. The

16

small expedition chose the rather grandiose name, American Bicentennial Expedition. Greatly to their credit they put two people on the summit, Chris Chandler and Bob Cormack.

Chris Chandler is a physician interested in high-altitude physiology, and I got together with him before the expedition to see if he would test the Medilog recorder high on Everest. When I first met Chris with his shoulder-length blond hair held in place by a bandana, beads around his neck, and sandals, I thought his chances of getting to the summit were not good. But as his performance on the mountain subsequently showed, this was an inaccurate judgment that no doubt reflected my middle-class prejudices. If I had known that he was going to climb so high, we would have done more intensive preliminary work on the Medilog recorder, but in the event he demonstrated that good data could be obtained up to about 7,300 meters (24,000 feet). In fact, we would probably have obtained an electrocardiogram from the summit if one of the electrode wires had not broken. This was valuable experience with a piece of equipment that became the backbone of many of the projects on the AMREE expedition.*

The notion gradually emerged of putting together a special dedicated medical research expedition to Everest. This was clearly extremely ambitious. For one thing, permission to climb Everest from the Nepalese side is given to only two or three groups each year, and all over the world top-class climbers are standing in line for the opportunity to attempt the world's highest mountain. Incidentally, the possibility of attempting the mountain from the north did not exist at this time. Relations with China were improving but expeditions to this strategically sensitive area were not yet permitted.

At about this time I offered to get some information on climbing oxygen equipment for the New Zealand expedition. As a result I talked to the Robertshaw Company in Los Angeles, which had developed the Robertshaw-Blume oxygen climbing equipment with Dr. Duane Blume of the Department of Biology at California State College at Bakersfield. Through this contact I met Duane, and it turned out that he too had been thinking about an expedition to do physiological research on Everest. Duane had been a member of the ill-fated International Everest Expedition in the spring of 1971. This was an ambitious undertaking with top climbers from several countries coming together to attempt the unclimbed southwest face of Everest and the West Ridge route. The expedition finally broke up amid a good deal of nationalistic squabbling. Duane had been given responsibility for the oxygen equipment of the expedition, and he had developed the Robertshaw-Blume design for this purpose.

*Tragically, Chris recently lost his life while attempting an oxygenless ascent of Kanchenjunga (8,598 meters, 28,207 feet).

Duane and I decided to pool our ideas. One of the most important early decisions was who would be climbing leader. We had no illusions about the cardinal importance of entrusting logistical decisions on the mountain to an expert climber. Any leading that I would do on the mountain would be from behind, as with Gilbert and Sullivan's Duke of Plaza-Toro:

In enterprise of martial kind, when there was any fighting
He led his regiment from behind—he found it less exciting

Fortunately Duane had become friendly with John Evans of Colorado who had been climbing leader of the 1971 International Expedition. John had shown remarkable poise in the face of extremely difficult circumstances, including the death of one of the climbers, appalling weather conditions, and a great deal of personal bickering. So we decided to invite John to take on the job of climbing leader of our expedition. There was a considerable delay while John did a lot of soul-searching about whether he was ready for a possible repeat of his 1971 experiences, but eventually he agreed. The American Medical Research Expedition to Everest could now begin serious planning.

3

PREPARATION

*"The idea of sending
a scientific expedition
to Everest is really deplorable"*[1]

When Dr. T. G. Longstaff, president of the Alpine Club, made this remark at a meeting of the Royal Geographical Society in London in 1938, he was voicing a popular view that no Everest expedition could properly combine the mixed objectives of climbing and science. Many would argue that this still holds. Climbing Mt. Everest is a logistical nightmare at the best of times. The mountain is situated over 100 miles from the nearest road in Nepal, and the mere transportation of tons of food and equipment to it is a challenge in itself. Some of the Nepalese authorities, although basically well intentioned, have acquired some of the worst bureaucratic attitudes of the British raj. Add to this the enormous complications of carrying out an ambitious scientific program, and the exercise can rapidly deteriorate into a morass of frustration.

The first hurdle to overcome is obtaining official permission to attempt to climb the mountain. The reason only three or four groups a year can attempt Everest via Nepal is that there are only two suitable climbing periods, immediately before and immediately after the summer monsoon, and the route cannot accommodate more than one large expedition at a time. There is now a third available slot in winter, but this is unattractive because of the low temperatures. There was, incidentally, another small expedition on the mountain with us, and with which we shared the route through the icefall, but this consisted of only two New Zealand climbers, Russell Brice and Paddy Freany, and two sherpas. Their base camp was a few hundred feet down the glacier from ours, and their two tents and tiny pile of equipment formed a striking contrast to our caravan of biblical proportions.

So in January 1978 we sent off our official application to His Majesty's Government of Nepal. Our letter duly followed the required protocol—"We are desirous of climbing the 8848 meter high Sagarmatha [the Nepalese name for Everest] Himalayan peak in the Kingdom of Nepal during either the Spring 1981, the Fall 1980, or the Fall 1981"—and gave assurances that we would abide by the mountaineering rules of His Majesty's Government. Prior to submitting this application we had applied for and received endorsement for the expedition from the American Alpine Club. This was essential if the Nepalese authorities were to consider our request. The application called for several pieces of information about which we had only foggy ideas, but we estimated the number of local porters to be 600, the cost of the expedition to be $350,000, and the total weight of equipment to be 36 tons. It was also necessary to name a Nepalese trekking agency for liaison between the expedition and the government. We chose Sherpa Cooperative Trekking Ltd., though we subsequently changed this to Mountain Travel, Nepal, because of their more extensive experience. This turned out to be a very satisfactory choice.

Nothing was heard for several months, and it was impossible to make definite plans without knowing when our slot would be (if ever). We knew that there were several other applications from various countries with the Ministry of Foreign Affairs in Kathmandu, and very likely there was diplomatic maneuvering by some governments who wanted to launch their first Everest expedition. By contrast, our pull with the State Department was nil. A second letter was sent reiterating our interest in the expedition, and pointing out that since the chief objective was to obtain a better understanding of the medical effects of living at high altitude, our findings might be of value to Nepalese living in the Himalayan regions. We also offered to include two Nepalese members in the expedition, suggesting that they might be doctors interested in relevant medical problems.

Finally on June 25, 1978 the hoped-for letter of permission arrived at the U.S. Embassy in Kathmandu, and was transmitted from there to us. The letter itself is something of a collector's item. The erratic behavior of the Nepalese typewriter contrasted greatly with the ponderous diplomatic sentiments—"His Majesty's Government of Nepal presents their compliments to the Embassy of the United States and begs to inform them that permission has been granted for the Medical Research Expedition to Everest for the post-monsoon period of 1981." This was great news. Planning for the expedition could begin in earnest.

We were a little disappointed that we were given the postmonsoon period. There was a general feeling that time was tighter in the fall, particularly as the Nepalese would not allow expeditions to enter the icefall prior to September 1. But by mid-October temperatures near the summit drop precipitously as winter approaches, and this period tends to be very windy. Thus there was a relatively short window in which the mountain could be climbed before conditions deteriorated. An additional hazard of the postmonsoon season is thought to be increased avalanche danger in the icefall, particularly if large amounts of snow have fallen during the monsoon. On the other hand, the premonsoon season has the disadvantage that an expedition can be cut short by an early monsoon, whereas the window for the postmonsoon season is perhaps more open-ended. Naturally the issue was completely academic as far as we were concerned, and we were lucky to have received permission at all.

In the summer of 1978 planning for the expedition accelerated rapidly. Duane Blume, John Evans, and myself met and formed a California corporation with ourselves as the three directors. One of the main advantages of this was that we could apply for nonprofit status, which meant that money donated to the expedition was tax-deductible. This was an important feature in attracting private donations. Forming a corporation also meant that if some disaster occurred during the expedition, our liability was limited.

During this period I wrote the first major grant application to support the expedition's scientific work. It was critical to get some money now to begin work on the scientific equipment. Although three years may seem a very long lead time, it soon evaporated as we started counting backward. For one thing, we hoped to pack and ship much of the equipment at the end of 1980 so that it could be carried into the Everest area prior to the monsoon. We needed to test some of the equipment in winter conditions, and this had to be done early in 1980. Furthermore, because the earliest date at which a grant application could be funded was mid-1979, we were already running on a tight schedule.

I sat down and composed a fifty-page grant application to the National Institutes of Health, the major government funding agency for medical research in the United States. The application outlined the reasons why it would be valuable to study the function of man during the extreme oxygen deprivation of high altitude, and described the research program in great detail. The budget was $182,000 for three years beginning in July 1979. Although this was not a particularly large sum for this type of application, it was important that the grant be funded at this time if the scientific part of the expedition was to get off the ground.

Grant applications to the NIH are dealt with in a democratic manner, and although this is one of the strengths of biomedical research in the United States, it can also be extremely frustrating. The application first goes to a Study Section composed of about fifteen scientists who are knowledgeable in the specific medical area. They discuss it in detail, sometimes requesting additional evaluations from other researchers who have particular expertise. At the end of the discussion the Study Section votes to approve or disapprove the application, and also assigns it a priority. To do this each member gives it a number between 100 and 500; the lower the number the higher the priority. All approved applications are subsequently ranked by priority number, and funds are assigned beginning with those with the highest priority, and going down until the funds for the year run out. Our application had one more hurdle to cross, a review by the National Heart, Lung and Blood Advisory Council. However, this group rarely changes a priority so that the decision of the "peer review" Study Section is critically important.

Our grant application had some very tough sledding. Although most of the Study Section was enthusiastic about the research, a minority group of three voted disapproval. The chief reasons they gave were that the project was too dangerous, and that government funds should not be used for such a hazardous enterprise. There were also some technical questions about the statistical significance of results on so few people. This last point did not bother me too much; one look at the back of the moon via an orbiting satellite was enough to see whether it was made of green cheese!

A vote of disapproval from several members of a Study Section is usually a death knell because their priority score is automatically 500, which drags down the overall priority score. So when I learned the outcome of the voting from the official report of the Study Section I was pessimistic, and as the year wore on and funding was not forthcoming, my pessimism deepened. However, a miracle happened in 1979. The National Heart, Lung and Blood Institute reported that just enough funds were available for the application to get through. This was extremely lucky, and was pivotal as far as developing the science was concerned. I believe that if this application had not been funded, we would have had to call off the expedition. It is worth adding that since mid-1980, NIH funding has become very much tighter, and certainly an application with the same priority score as ours would not be funded at the present time. Thus this was one of a series of lucky events that kept recurring throughout the story of this expedition.

With the money in hand we could now set about the serious business of designing the experiments and equipment. Most of this would be done in the respiratory physiology laboratories at the University of California at San Diego. But a new problem arose: we needed additional technical staff with very special qualifications. Once again providence intervened and the story is a strange one.

One of our laboratory technicians was having dinner at a vegetarian restaurant in San Diego when he got into a conversation with the waiter. He was considerably taken aback to learn that this young man was a newly qualified M.D. who was waiting on tables to make ends meet. "Why don't you come and see Dr. West," he said. "He might be able to find something more productive for you to do." So Dr. Karl Maret made an appointment to see me.

Our laboratory virtually never has funds to take somebody on at short notice because the budgeting is done several years in advance. But because we had just received the grant to develop scientific equipment for the expedition, I had my eyes open for someone trained in medical instrumentation with some experience at high altitudes. However, when Karl Maret walked in, my face fell. His curly hair hung down to his shoulders, there were beads around his neck, and he came slopping in with sandaled feet. The most striking feature was his eyes which had an excited look that I do not associate with a science laboratory.

Karl's story was that he had recently graduated from the University of Toronto. However, he had become disenchanted with conventional medicine during his last year or so at medical school, and instead of taking the traditional route of a residency after graduation, he had joined a holistic medicine group called the Fashioners of Manas. Their belief was that healthy living came about as a consequence of meditation, vegetarian food, music, and dance. The organization was in financial difficulties, and Karl was obliged to spend some of his time working as a waiter.

On the face of it, Karl's background looked very unpromising at best. But as we continued talking I found myself surprised. When asked whether he had any experience in medical instrumentation, Karl replied that he had earned a master's degree in bioengineering at the University of Toronto prior to having received his medical degree. Furthermore, he had worked on a high-altitude project carried out by Dr. Charles Houston on Mt. Logan. Thus in spite of his unconventional appearance, he had ideal qualifications.

Karl took the job, and he subsequently proved to be one of the most valuable members of our expedition. He was responsible for much of the innovative equipment design, and indeed, without his participation the expedition would have been entirely different. But the two sides of Karl's personality always remained in evidence. I could never get used to the fact that a conversation on some technical aspect of transistors might progress to a discussion of levitation; his dietary peculiarities and harp playing at the high camps were a source of endless jokes. But as an electronic engineer Karl was a genius who was responsible for much of the scientific success of the expedition.

In the fall of 1978 the job of choosing the members of the expedition began in earnest. Duane Blume, John Evans, and I discussed the design of the expedition extensively, and we decided that we needed three kinds of people. The first were the climbers whose job was to put in the route and get to the summit. But not any top-class climbers would do. These had to be people who believed in the primary scientific purpose of the expedition, and were prepared to support it. This meant specifically that if a conflict arose between scientific and mountaineering objectives, science would come first. In these discussions Duane and I were tremendously encouraged by the attitude of John Evans, the climbing leader. Clearly, his stance was going to be critical for determining the relationship between the climbers and the expedition objectives. As climbing leader, John would be responsible for choosing the climbers, and for sounding them out on their reactions to conflicting situations. For example, getting all the science equipment up to Camp 2 would delay route-finding on the upper part of the mountain, and thus make the expedition more vulnerable to the deteriorating weather of late October. Would a particular climber accept this? John was adamant that science had to have first priority, and he never wavered on this point throughout many difficult decisions on the mountain. The scientific success of the expedition owes a great deal to him.

Actually, John's own credentials as a scientist were not inconsiderable. He obtained B.S. and Master's degrees in geological engineering from the South Dakota School of Mines. He had worked at NASA's Johnson Space Center in Houston, Texas, studying rocks brought back from the moon. He had also carried out geological research in Antarctica, and while there had been a member of a team that made first ascents of several peaks for which they received the La Gorce medal of the National Geographic Society.

John made a striking impression on anyone who met him. With his shock of fair hair, brilliant blue eyes, and arms and shoulders bulging with muscles he was the archetype of the Hollywood good guy. He was an instant success with my children, Joanna and Robert, aged 7 and 9 at the time, when he described how he used to wrestle alligators when he worked for a period in a reptile park in his college days. He gave a riveting account of how the unfortunate animal was carefully stalked and then immobilized by grasping its jaws. As can be imagined, my children's eyes were out on stalks.

Since 1971 John had been Program Director of the Outward Bound School in Denver. His work there involved taking young people on challenging treks into the Rocky Mountains where a knowledge of mountain craft and the ability to handle various personalities were equally important. A feature of the Outward Bound program is that a particular party of young people often has a very broad cross-section including some from correctional facilities, and some from wealthy homes. John's knowledge of human nature and his ability to deal with difficult interpersonal situations with tact were valuable attributes on the expedition. I cannot think of a better climbing leader for our complex organization.

Duane Blume's qualifications for the expedition were also outstanding. He had obtained his Ph.D. from the University of California at Berkeley in 1964 under Dr. Nello Pace, who is well known in the area of environmental physiology, and who kindly agreed to serve on our scientific Advisory Committee. Several other prominent scientists also agreed to help us in this way, including Dr. Charles Houston, D. B. Dill, Thomas Hornbein, Dr. Robert Grover from the University of Colorado, and Dr. John Severinghaus from the University of California at San Francisco. Duane had then spent several years, first as a postdoctoral fellow and later as assistant director, at the University of California's high-altitude White Mountain Research Station near Bishop, California. Here he had shown himself to be a productive scientist and a good manager. Since 1972 he had been chairman of biology at California State College at Bakersfield. As expedition treasurer he was able to arrange for all the expedition accounts to go through the College Foundation with the great advantages of professional accounting.

Duane's intimate knowledge of expedition oxygen equipment was a considerable asset. He had designed the Robertshaw-Blume equipment for the 1971 International Everest Expedition, and he took on the responsibility for oxygen on our expedition. His area of research was the biochemical and metabolic changes in the body at high altitude, and this nicely complemented my own interests in the cardio-respiratory area. He had useful climbing experience; he was one of the only two members of the expedition (John Evans was the other) who had previously been through the Khumbu icefall. Added to all this, Duane has an engaging personality and an infectious sense of humor that enlivens any camp. His role in the expedition was pivotal, and he can be justly proud of its success.

The choice of the five climbers (six with John Evans) was principally made by John, though each one was discussed with Duane and myself. A very early choice was Glenn Porzak, an attorney from Denver, whom John had known for some time. Glenn was a very strong climber with extensive experience in North America, Europe, South America, and the Himalaya. In 1978 he had led an expedition to Manaslu and at that time had incidentally shown one of the advantages of having an attorney in the party. During the approach to the mountain, a truck carrying some of the porters overturned and, tragically, several were killed. The expedition was sued for an enormous sum of money and Glenn took on the task of legal defense. Although the case was ultimately settled out of court, Glenn's versatility and enterprise as a lawyer in a foreign country were dramatically shown. And the fact that he was chairman of the Expeditions Committee of the American Alpine Club was also useful since our expedition had both endorsement and sponsorship from this prestigious organization. As an expedition companion, Glenn had a quick wit and lively personality.

Jeff Lowe and Michael Weis were two friends of John's from Colorado. Each had impressive qualifications. Jeff is one of the country's top ice climbers, and his book *The Ice Experience* is well known. He is a professional mountaineer who divides his time between being a guide and running a successful family business that makes mountaineering equipment and clothing. Jeff's gentle, sympathetic personality belies his drive on a mountain, and he was a key member of the climbing group. He was also completely supportive of the scientific objectives.

Mike Weis is a self-employed mountain guide with considerable experience in North America, South America, and the French Alps, though this was his first visit to the Himalaya. He was well read, and an entertaining conversationalist on a great variety of issues; he also took charge of recorded music at Base Camp, and his knowledge of the various varieties of rock music made me feel very square.

David Jones is a Canadian from British Columbia who was a graduate student in physical geography at the time of the expedition. His extensive climbing experience included expeditions to Makalu in 1974 and Manaslu four years later. He had an almost boyish enthusiasm and drive, and was particularly interested in the medical research. Together with Brownie Schoene and Duane Blume he shouldered the large and thankless job of organizing the food. His hallmark was an enormous jug that he used as a cup to consume vast quantities of fluid. Davey had a prodigious appetite to match, and his performance at mealtimes was an indictment to all who were bored with the food.

Chris Kopczynski was the last climber to join the expedition, but he proved to be one of the strongest. A building contractor in a large family business in Spokane, his very extensive climbing experience included an attempt on Makalu. He had also climbed with John Evans in the U.S.S.R. on Pik Lenin. Chris sometimes gave the impression that he preferred his own company to that of a noisy group, but his enormous drive and determination paid handsome dividends.

Although the climbers were primarily chosen for their role in route-finding and summit bids, they took part in the physiological measurements, and they were all trained to carry out the scientific experiments at extreme altitudes. A feature of the expedition was the close relationships between the climbers and scientists, and the climber's interest in the research program. When a severe snowstorm confined everybody to Base Camp in the early part of September, we had a series of informal afternoon seminars about the scientific program, and the climbers were always there. In fact, they had their turn to give a seminar on the physics of snow conditions after the big avalanche on September 9 when the windblast rocked Base Camp and we subsequently moved most of the tents.

The next group of expedition members were the climbing scientists. This was a critical group, and the idea was unique to this expedition. Since the primary objective was to make measurements of human physiology at extreme altitudes, we needed scientists who were very strong climbers. In the event, all six members of this group were M.D.s with an interest in high-altitude physiology—in fact, a couple of them had already done a good deal of scientific research in high-altitude medicine—and several could have qualified as members of the climbing group with no difficulty.

The first in this group was Steven Boyer. Steve had obtained his M.D. from the University of Colorado four years previously, and was employed as an emergency room physician. (This is a favorite occupation for serious climbers. Two other climbing scientists did the same, the reason being that the job allows you to take off for several months at a time.) Steve had previously obtained an M.S. in geology, and had written several articles on rock weathering. He is intensely competitive, continually competing against himself; typically he would time himself going from one camp to another. In addition to extensive climbing experience in North America, South America, New Zealand, and even Antarctica, he had finished seventh in the Pike's Peak marathon four years earlier. This remarkable race is up to and down from the summit of Pike's Peak at an elevation of 4,300 meters (14,110 feet)! Steve's chief research interest was nutrition and body weight, and he collaborated a good deal with Duane Blume on these studies.

David Graber has an M.D. from Baylor University, and is also an emergency room physician. He had amassed extensive climbing experience in North America, Iran, and Nepal. Although he had not had much opportunity to do research, he had extensive experience as an expedition physician, and his medical opinion was much sought after. I certainly felt confident when he treated a nasty infection of my right elbow during my period at Base Camp. Dave is unusually tall, and his size 16 boot became a minor expedition legend; he was usually referred to as "Big D."

Peter Hackett was one of our most knowledgeable members on high-altitude medical problems. His M.D. was from the University of Illinois, and he spends some time each year at a medical clinic in Pheriche, a small Nepalese village two or three days' walk from the Everest Base Camp. As a consequence he has probably seen more trekkers with acute mountain sickness than anyone else in the world, and he has published a small book on the subject. He has an intimate knowledge of the sherpas in that area, and has adopted two sherpa boys who attend the Hillary School in Khumjung. This school was erected by the 1960–61 expedition, and it is one of the focal points of Ed Hillary's close involvement with the Sola Khumbu region where most of the sherpas live. Peter has climbed extensively in Nepal and elsewhere.

Christopher Pizzo is a pathologist who obtained his M.D. from Indiana University in 1976. Another very successful competitor in the Pike's Peak marathon (he also finished in the top ten), he had climbed in North and South America, India, Nepal, and the U.S.S.R. He could easily have merited a place as a regular climber, and as will become evident, he played a crucial role in the expedition's scientific success.

Frank Sarnquist is an assistant professor of anesthesia at Stanford University Medical School. He has had extensive climbing experience in several countries, and has been expedition physician to many climbing groups. As designated team physician he was responsible for putting together the medical supplies. We recognized very early on that with ten M.D.s on the expedition there would be no shortage of medical opinions, and it was clearly essential to define the responsibility for medical decisions. Frank also did a great job training the sherpa cooks in hygiene, which doubtless paid dividends as we had relatively few gastrointestinal ailments. One of Frank's monuments was an enormous water purifier that some unfortunate sherpa lugged all the way to Base Camp.

The group of climbing scientists was completed by Robert (Brownie) Schoene, M.D., a member of the Division of Respiratory Diseases at the University of Washington in Seattle. With several scientific papers on respiratory physiology to his credit, he was one of the group's strongest scientists. An experienced climber, he too was a competitive marathon runner. Stunningly handsome and a natural charmer, Brownie was always the first to get a big smile from the aircraft stewardesses.

Initially, we saw the chief role of the climbing scientists as carrying out research at Camp 5 on the South Col, and attaching scientific recorders to the climbers before they left that camp for the summit. In fact, during the recruitment negotiations, John Evans, Duane Blume, and I repeatedly stressed the fact that the climbing scientists would probably not have an opportunity to go to the summit. We believed that if they joined the expedition with this expectation, they might not be willing to devote the necessary energies to the scientific measurements. In retrospect, this was naive. Getting to the summit of Everest is so tough that an expedition will probably need everybody who is fit enough to make a summit bid. Indeed, as the expedition wore on, the distinction between climbers and climbing scientists became increasingly blurred. The final irony was when two of the three Americans to reach the summit were in fact climbing scientists!

The final group was the scientists. They were generally older and had had some research experience at high altitudes. Sukhamay Lahiri, Ph.D., was from Calcutta via Oxford University, and is now professor of physiology at the University of Pennsylvania. Together with Jim Milledge and myself, he was on the Himalayan Scientific and Mountaineering Expedition of 1960–61, and he has published extensively in the area of respiratory physiology. He has an international reputation for his research on the control of breathing at high altitudes. Fluent in Hindi, he could always clarify a point with the sherpas if the usual patois was inadequate, though this was rarely the case. Larry (as most of us called him) was responsible for most of the research program at the Base Camp laboratory. However, toward the end of October he made a brief excursion through the icefall to Camp 2 to prove to everybody (but chiefly to himself, I suspect) that he could do it!

James Milledge, M.D., is a scientific staff member with the Medical Research Council at Northwick Park in London. He has been on several medical research expeditions to Nepal, and has an extensive list of publications in the area of high-altitude physiology. He was the most experienced climber among the scientists. In addition, as "our man in England," Jim was a key person in the planning stages of the expedition. The two stationary bicycles that we used for exercise measurements were constructed in the machine shop at Northwick Park; we wanted them to be identical to the very satisfactory bicycles used on the 1960–61 expedition, and the original was available there. Jim also played a critical role in getting the oxygen equipment ready. Although the special high-pressure tanks were bought in California, they had to be filled in England because of regulations on the transportation of oxygen at very high pressure. There were innumerable delays because of faulty valves and the like, which put the expedition in jeopardy at one stage, and Jim's contribution here was crucial. Jim is a close personal friend of mine and we shared a tent during the periods at Base Camp and Camp 2. His cheerfulness and general good sense were a great support when the going got tough.

Richard Peters was the youngest member of the expedition, being only 25 at the time. He had recently graduated from Stanford, and was in the process of applying to medical school. In 1979 we gave him a temporary job as a laboratory technician while we were preparing the scientific equipment, and he was so able and valuable in this area that we offered him a place on the expedition. Working closely with Karl Maret he did a magnificent job of keeping the equipment in working order and helping with the running of the experiments. Initially we thought that Rick would remain at Base Camp, but his technical know-how and physical toughness were so impressive that he was one of the first scientists to go to Camp 2 where he and Jim Milledge set up the laboratory.

Robert Winslow, M.D., is a blood physiologist who has studied high-altitude physiology in the Peruvian Andes. He has an impressive list of publications. Bob had never climbed before, but his performance in the icefall and elsewhere was outstanding. He worked closely with Michele Samaja, Ph.D., from Milan, who had taken part in a previous Italian Scientific Himalayan expedition in 1976. Mickey had worked with Bob at the National Institutes of Health in Bethesda, Maryland, and was an experienced rock climber in the Italian Dolomites.

The only other American on the expedition was Rodney Korich, Base Camp manager. Rodney had been a member of several previous expeditions to Nepal, chiefly as manager. He is a travel agent, and he helped to arrange the air transportation of both personnel and equipment. He also cleared a large sea shipment through Indian Customs at a critical time. At one stage it looked as if one of the expedition members from the United States would have to make a special trip to Calcutta for this purpose, and the fact that Rodney was already there on another job saved us a lot of expense.

One feature of the personnel selection that occasionally required defending was the absence of women. The simple answer is that unfortunately there are very few women trained in the area of high-altitude physiology. And although there are a number of strong women climbers, the strongest climbers are men. But I would be less than candid if I claimed that these were the only reasons. We felt that the presence of one or two women might create additional tensions that an expedition of this complexity could ill afford. Some will brand our attitude as ultraconservative or even chauvinistic, but I believe that the results of the expedition help to vindicate our decision.

The recruiting of climbers and scientists took place over many months, and it was not until late 1980 that the final decisions were made. We were very careful in our selection; all the expedition members were previously known to Duane, John, or myself. In addition, after we had determined someone's climbing and/or scientific qualifications, we gave a great deal of thought to whether that person would fit in with our group. The tensions of living at close quarters in a hostile environment are obviously such that a premium is placed on how well someone can fit in with a group. Whether it was by good luck or good management (or a combination of both), the final outcome exceeded expectations. There were very few personal conflicts, and virtually everybody parted good friends with everybody else. In fact, while expeditions generally have a reputation for breaking up families, causing divorces and other personal crises, ours was exceptional in that several single members got married shortly after, and the potential climbing population for the 1990s increased by at least five!

While the selection of climbers and scientists was going on there was intense activity in many other areas. The preparation and testing of scientific equipment was going full steam ahead. One of the largest projects here was the design and construction of the rigid laboratory hut. We originally planned to take this up to Camp 2 but later decided to substitute a lighter semirigid structure. The hut did sterling service at Base Camp. It was designed by Douglas Deeds, a boat designer in San Diego, and was constructed of panels of plastic foam (Klegecell) sandwiched between layers of Kevlar, a material with an extremely high tensile strength. The materials were donated by the manufacturers (American Klegecell Corp., and E. I. Dupont Inc.), which was typical of the generous support that we received from industry

The panels were small enough to be carried by a porter, and once they reached Base Camp they were bolted together to form a rectangular-shaped laboratory. In March 1980 Karl Maret and Rick Peters managed to get the hut to the summit of Mammoth Mountain in northern California by snowcat, and it was extensively tested there over a period of several days. At the same time measurements were made on the solar panels that we planned to use to generate electricity at Base Camp and Camp 2.

One of the largest obstacles to be overcome was raising the money. In addition to the usual costs of food, climbing equipment, porters, air fares, and dozens of unforeseen extras, the science component was very expensive. The initial grant from the National Institutes of Health was essentially seed money; most of it was used to buy or build equipment. Although we managed to get much of the equipment donated or lent to us by industry, there was still a great deal of money needed. Our rough estimate was about $500,000.

In the summer of 1978, shortly after we received permission from the Nepalese government to climb, we started serious fund-raising. Initially we thought we could raise a substantial amount by sending proposals to various foundations and corporations. After all, the first medical scientific expedition to Everest should have some pizzazz. We even paid a public relations firm about $2,000 to supply us with lists of names and help with the preparation

31

of the letters, but this proved to be money down the drain. It rapidly became apparent that without some kind of personal contact, there was just too much competition for the charitable dollar.

Over the course of the next three years fund-raising was never far from our minds, and it was always a depressing subject. All of us made fruitless tries to plead our case to tycoons, but gradually we made progress. Duane Blume put together a brochure describing the plans for the expedition, and I initiated a series of newsletters. We missed no opportunity to talk to the press, television, and radio, and there were innumerable telephone calls, visits to important people, and generally making the rounds, cap in hand. Instinctively I felt much of this was demeaning, and certainly some of my scientific colleagues sneered at our Madison Avenue approach. But we needed a great deal of money, and times were tough. The list of donors to the expedition (bless their hearts) is in Appendix E.

We had one unusual advantage. Because of the scientific objectives of the expedition we could make formal applications to various large granting agencies. A big shot in the arm was a grant of $35,000 from the Committee for Research and Exploration of the National Geographic Society. Here we had a great deal of valuable advice from Barry Bishop, who had been with National Geographic for many years, and whom I knew from the 1960–61 expedition. This was followed by grants of $73,000 to Sukhamay Lahiri from the National Heart, Lung and Blood Institute for his work on the control of ventilation, and another of $31,000 to Duane Blume from the National Science Foundation for his project on metabolic changes at high altitudes. A lucky break was when Servier Laboratories of Paris agreed to support a project to study the effect of a new drug on sleep at high altitudes (just before we left for Nepal they decided not to go ahead with the project, but we had already spent the money, so they graciously left things as they were!). Additional grants came from the American Alpine Club, the American Lung Association, the Explorers Club, the U.S. Army Medical Research and Development Command, and the Chancellor's Associates at UCSD. Each expedition member contributed $1,000 as part of his agreement.

We also received some financial help from Mountain Travel USA who organized two treks to our Base Camp while we were on the mountain. The leaders were Charles Houston, M.D., and Gil Roberts, M.D., who was the chief medical officer on the 1963 American Everest expedition. Both treks were specially designed for people interested in high-altitude medical problems, and were limited to fifteen members. They arrived at Base Camp in mid-October and each had their share of incidents en route, though most participants reported that the long walk was a memorable though sometimes challenging experience. A portion of the fee went directly to our expedition, and we were grateful to Mountain Travel, Charlie Houston, and Gil Roberts for their help.

In spite of the grant money and the corporate and individual donations, it was clear that the expedition was going to be substantially in the red when it took off for Nepal. Fortunately, Duane Blume persuaded the College Foundation at Bakersfield to make us a loan to be paid back at the end of the expedition. Once we got to Nepal there were a number of unexpected expenses, and it did not help us sleep to know that we were going to return some $30,000 in debt! However, the eventual success of the expedition enabled us to cover this within six months of our return.

Sometimes I am asked what the expedition cost, but it is impossible to come up with an accurate figure because so much of the equipment and supplies were donated. My best guess is $500,000, and I am astonished that some people think this unduly expensive. It was a bargain bearing in mind the extensive scientific program accomplished. As I write this I am heavily involved in a big experiment to fly on the NASA Spacelab 4. This experiment will cost at least ten times as much, and we shall be lucky if we get one-tenth of the data that we obtained on the expedition!

There were a host of other chores. John Evans took charge of selecting and ordering the specialized clothing and climbing equipment. Much of this came from Colorado where some of the big suppliers are located, and he was greatly helped by Jeff Lowe, Mike Weis, and Glenn Porzak. Some of the equipment and clothing was donated, and much else was provided at a reduced price. Individual expedition members were responsible for buying most of their own clothing, but a large expense was providing high-altitude clothing for the 42 sherpas who were employed by the expedition above Base Camp. The Nepalese mountaineering regulations set out in detail what clothing should be supplied for these sherpas and this represents a very substantial expedition expense. In fact this is one of the perks for many sherpas because frequently they do not wear the clothing at all during the expedition but sell it at the end.

Davey Jones, Brownie Schoene, and Duane Blume took on the enormous job of ordering food. With 65 mouths to feed at Base Camp and above (21 climbers and scientists plus 42 sherpas and 2 liaison officers) for about two months, the logistics are mind-boggling. Some food can be bought in Kathmandu, and a few fresh vegetables can be obtained at villages a few days from Base Camp, but most of the food had to be acquired in the U.S. and shipped across. Because of our financial stringency, strenuous efforts were made to have much of the food donated. We were successful, but the disadvantage of this approach was lack of balance—there were exotic delicacies such as caviar and smoked shrimp, but a definite shortage of canned beef. However, I am glad to report that we never had to resort to the Spartan attitudes of some expeditions, notably those led by H. W. Tilman. He described a Tibetan mail runner on one of his treks who was reduced to boiling his shirt in order to make a cup of tea. On the other hand, Tilman showed considerable enterprise in living off the land. On one day during the 1935 British Everest Reconnaissance Expedition a party of four ate 140 eggs!

John Evans now started work on a detailed climbing plan. It is often said that an 8,000-meter peak cannot be climbed unless at least three things go right: weather, health, and logistics. Indeed, climbing a mountain like Everest is rather like waging a war; *everything* has to be in the right place at the right time. The logistics are so complicated that Chris Bonington in his fine book *Everest—The Hard Way* describes a computer program for climbing Everest. After reading it I wrote to the man in England who had put it together, and actually succeeded in getting it to run on one of the laboratory computers, but I cannot claim that we made much practical use of it.

Duane Blume took on the responsibility of arranging transportation for all the equipment and supplies. Our plan was to send the bulk of this by sea from Los Angeles to Calcutta, and then overland to Kathmandu. We hoped that the loads would arrive in Nepal in time to be carried in to the Everest region in the spring of 1981 prior to the monsoon. This would have two advantages. First, there would be less danger of the supplies being damaged by rain. More important, it would lessen the logistic difficulties of carrying all the 20 tons or so of material from Kathmandu to the Everest Base Camp with the main body of the expedition in August. This turned out to be a very wise decision; we encountered great difficulties in carrying in the 300 loads of essential supplies in August because of a severe shortage of porters.

Duane also worked on the oxygen equipment. We had a number of discussions about the best type of equipment to use. The chief contenders were the very simple bag-and-mask arrangement originally designed by Hornbein, and used successfully on the American 1963 expedition, versus the more sophisticated Robertshaw-Blume design that Duane had developed for the 1971 International Everest Expedition. Although the latter was more sophisticated and efficient in terms of the amount of oxygen used, many climbers preferred the simplicity of the Hornbein design. It is immediately apparent to the user whether the system is operating properly because he can see the bag inflating and deflating with each breath. By contrast, there is no direct evidence that the special valve of the Robertshaw-Blume equipment that mixes oxygen with air is working correctly. We ended up taking both types of equipment, but the climbers generally preferred the Hornbein design, and all five summiters eventually chose it.

Preparations reached a climax toward the end of 1980 as mountains of food, clothing, and climbing equipment accumulated at Bakersfield, and the science equipment and supplies converged on La Jolla. During December the piles were sorted and resorted and placed in special waterproof containers, each weighing 30 kilograms (66 pounds). Each container would be one porterload in Nepal. In all, over 380 porterloads were prepared for shipment on the freighter *President Tyler*, which set sail for Calcutta from Los Angeles on January 24, 1981. This represented over 10 tons of equipment and supplies, which would be combined with another 10 tons to be purchased in Kathmandu. The shipment arrived in Calcutta in March where Rodney Korich cleared it through Indian Customs and arranged for it to be transported by truck to Kathmandu. There, Mountain Travel, our local agents, arranged for the containers to be carried in to the village of Khunde near Everest where the loads were stored in houses and watched over by sherpas to await our arrival in late August.

There were the inevitable crises. At the last minute we found that the propane we needed for heating the two laboratories could not be shipped with the rest of the supplies because of its flammability. It had to wait for another freighter, and had still not arrived in Kathmandu when we began our trek into Base Camp in early August. However, it eventually showed up, and worked well although we had great difficulty in starting the laboratory heater at Camp 2. Finally we accepted the fact that it was as oxygen-deprived as we were, and we filled it with climbing oxygen to fire it up.

We were flattered and encouraged to receive four official documents showing that others thought all the trouble was worthwhile. One was a letter from the White House with an elegant embossed letterhead. President Reagan extended his best wishes for success: "This project is unique in focusing on medical research as the primary concern of an expedition with summit aspirations. The results of your research may have implications for all of mankind and that is the best tradition of pioneering efforts in medicine. The goals and aspirations of your mission capture the imagination of our people and symbolize the drive for accomplishment that is the heart of the American spirit."

We also received a very supportive letter from the governor of California, Edmund G. Brown, Jr., and a proclamation from the governor of Colorado, Richard D. Lamm. Finally, we received a resolution from the California legislature with lots of preliminary Whereas paragraphs and ending with a nice fat Resolution.

The final stage of the preparations took place in May 1981 when the members of the expedition came to La Jolla for baseline testing and training. Eighteen climbers and scientists took part in these tests (the only participants not present were the two overseas members, Michele Samaja from Italy and Jim Milledge from England). The busy program occupied most of the latter half of May. First, everybody had a full physical examination including electrocardiograms and blood tests. Then a series of exercise studies was done on each member so that the data obtained at sea level could subsequently be compared with measurements made at high altitudes. Various blood samples were taken for biochemical measurements, again for high-altitude comparison.

One morning was devoted to a battery of psychometric tests carried out by Robert Reed and his collaborators at the La Jolla Veterans Administration Hospital. These tests had been designed by Dr. Brenda Townes of the University of Washington, in collaboration with Dr. Tom Hornbein. Tom, who is chairman of the Department of Anesthesiology there, is well known in climbing circles as one of the first five Americans to reach the summit of Everest during the highly successful 1963 expedition, and he agreed to be one of the six members of the Scientific Advisory Committee of the present expedition. An abbreviated series of these psychological tests was conducted at high altitude, and the whole battery was repeated at the end of the expedition in Kathmandu. The results were extremely interesting—they clearly showed that some impairment of brain function had occurred as a result of the expedition (see Chapter 8).

Finally, we devoted several afternoons to familiarization with the scientific equipment, particularly for the climbers who were being trained to carry out measurements above 8,000 meters. This went extremely well; those climbers who had not had any previous exposure to the equipment generally felt that all the measurements were feasible and that they could fit them in without too much interruption to their normal climbing schedule.

One of the best features of these preexpedition studies was the opportunity for expedition members to meet each other. Almost everyone stayed in a spare room in our house adjacent to the La Jolla campus, and there were early morning runs, a barbecue on the beach, and a good deal of spirited competition to see who had the highest oxygen consumption on the stationary bicycle.

These two weeks did more than give us baseline scientific data. Many people met other expedition members for the first time, and we had a chance to size each other up. In some ways we were a very heterogeneous group for an attempt on Mt. Everest, and there was a good deal of melding to be done. This got off to a good start in La Jolla and continued during the long walk into Base Camp.

4

APPROACH

---

*"A prodigious white fang excrescent
from the jaw of the world"*[1]

An overloaded bus careens across the road to avoid a cow, two saffron-robed monks walk past the woman squatting on the pavement selling betel nuts, a pedal rickshaw bowls along with an important-looking white-suited government official, a small boy relieves himself of an unformed stool in the shade of an elaborately carved Hindu temple. In short, Kathmandu.

Duane Blume, John Evans, Rodney Korich, Rick Peters, and I had arrived after the long flight from Seattle. We traveled on Royal Thai Airlines because they gave us a good deal on air freight, and we had spent the night in Bangkok. The predawn taxi ride from the hotel to the airport was memorable; the frangipani lei hanging from the driver's mirror gave out a heavy tropical scent, and the dawn really did come up like thunder.

We had our first meeting with Rodney Korich at the Bangkok airport. He was full of bounce, somewhat garishly dressed with a cap that said "Colorado" in iridescent colors, and obviously looking forward to the battle of getting our stuff through Customs. We were not traveling lightly. Some eyebrows had gone up at the Seattle airport when we assembled twenty-six pieces of "personal baggage," some almost too heavy to lift, but Royal Thai Airlines looked the other way, and there was no charge. We were bringing last-minute items of fragile scientific equipment that we wanted to keep our eyes on.

The send-off at Seattle airport was enlivened by a press and television conference arranged by Royal Thai Airlines and we were given blue T-shirts proclaiming that Thai flew to the roof of the world. Prior to this there was a more private ceremony in the Men's Room where Brownie Schoene gave John Evans a shot of gamma globulin to ward off hepatitis, after borrowing a dime for accommodations.

Our plane made a hair-raising landing at Kathmandu airport in low cloud after one aborted approach (the airport is ringed by hills), and memories of this exotic city flooded back to me. Although I had last been there twenty years ago, it was immediately familiar. The sideways shake of the head meaning yes, the thunderous hawking, and the special way of clearing a nostril made an instant impression. Rodney assembled the bags, and chatted away to the Customs people. I gave him $100 to expedite matters, and never saw the money again, but it must have been well spent because we had no trouble. (I cannot remember how this particular expense was justified when I finally reckoned up our expenditures for the accounting department at the University of California at the end of the expedition.)

We were extricated from the airport chaos, and driven to the Hotel Malla where we stayed in style. In the afternoon we went out to Mountain Travel, the local trekking firm handling our affairs, to meet Bobby Chettri who immediately impressed us as personable and capable. His office was seven or eight times as large as mine at UCSD, and he seemed to have an unlimited supply of clerks to fetch and carry.

Mountain Travel is one of the oldest and best-known trekking agencies in Nepal. It was started by Colonel James (Jimmy) Roberts who was with the British Army there, and who was largely responsible for opening up the country to trekkers. A trekking agency performs a critically important role for an expedition. It is the interface between the expedition and the government of Nepal, and it makes arrangements for the lowland porters and high-altitude sherpas. Mountain Travel was efficient and knowledgeable, and they were an enormous asset to our expedition.

We had ten days in Kathmandu before setting off on the trek to Base Camp, and these were dominated by the Nepalese Customs. Import duties in Nepal are outrageous; presumably this is where the government raises a sizable portion of its budget. We had air freighted much of the scientific equipment from the U.S. either because it was relatively fragile or because we needed to work with it in La Jolla until June. In spite of our advantageous arrangement with Royal Thai Airlines, the freight bill was over $13,000, and the Nepalese wanted

27 percent of that, or $3,500, in duty! This was in addition to duty on the value of the equipment itself.

Most expeditions try to counter the absurd import duties by putting ridiculously low valuations on the equipment. We routinely reduced the nominal value to one-tenth, and in the case of some of the expensive scientific equipment, to one-hundredth. For example, an oximeter which looked like an overgrown radio with a few dials and knobs would have its value declared as $100 whereas it cost us $10,000! Even so the duty was staggering and we spent a good deal of time looking for ways to reduce it.

It occurred to us that we might reduce the cost by guaranteeing that large pieces of equipment would be reexported. This involved trotting around to the U.S. Embassy, the Ministry of Tourism, the Ministry of Foreign Affairs, and the Customs Department. The usual frustrations of waiting around government departments were magnified a hundred-fold here by the apparently unlimited number of petty clerks. When we finally got permission to move the scientific equipment out of Customs we were devastated to find that the air shipment had been badly damaged. Rick Peters spent a couple of hours searching the floor of the Customs shed looking for bits of the stationary bicycles, and of course we were apprehensive about the delicate electronic black boxes. However, the final outcome was a happy one—the bicycles were finally assembled intact at Base Camp, and most of the electronics survived the trip, though it needed constant love and care from Karl Maret and Rick Peters.

Various crises arose and were resolved. Our walkie-talkie radios for communicating between camps had illegal frequencies, but this was solved simply by saying they didn't. (In fact, the frequencies allocated by the Nepalese were inappropriate for the sort of radio links we needed.) Our large shipment of propane for heating that had been delayed in Los Angeles because of its flammability was either in Calcutta or somewhere between there and Kathmandu—no one had any idea. There were unexpected expenses, and we suddenly found ourselves short of $10,000, but Mountain Travel generously covered that until we could cable for more money. We needed a tank of liquid nitrogen at Base Camp to freeze blood samples, and this looked like an insurmountable obstacle. The very cold liquid was sometimes available in Nepal, but we were out of luck this time. But even if it could be obtained, it was impracticable to carry it in by porters because so much would be lost by evaporation en route. We considered flying it in, but fixed-wing aircraft could not land anywhere near the mountains in the monsoon, and the only helicopters in Nepal belonged to the army; they flew for civilians only when there was a medical emergency. Finally we cabled Karl Maret who was coming in later asking him to pick up some liquid nitrogen in Calcutta, and I wrote a formal request to the Nepalese Army for the use of one of their helicopters to fly it into the Everest area. Somehow, this plan worked.

Unexpected delays were frequent. We had planned a big program of work for July 31 when we suddenly found, just the evening before, that it was a national holiday. The reason was a partial eclipse of the sun (we didn't see it—the sun had shone for only about 10 minutes during our whole period in Kathmandu and much of the time the monsoon rains were pelting down). The Hindus regard the eclipse as a resurgence of evil over good, and by tradition everyone goes down to the river to wash. This has to be a good thing because washing facilities in Kathmandu are very poor and certainly not overused. However a note in my diary reminds me that I did see an enterprising man washing his car using a large muddy puddle of water left by a monsoon downpour.

Between crises it was nice to go back to the Malla Hotel with its old world, Eastern elegance. Because we were in the middle of the monsoon, there were very few tourists, so often there were more waiters for dinner than guests. The curries were excellent (my period of living in London had left me addicted to them) although the beer was exorbitant at $3.00 a bottle. But everything was done in great style, and one could hardly imagine a greater contrast to the three months to come.

One of the problems that needed sorting out was how to deal with expedition mail. Here we had a great deal of help from Elizabeth Hawley, a remarkable American woman who has lived in Kathmandu for many years. In addition to working with Tiger Tops Ltd., a subsidiary of Mountain Travel, Nepal, and being the local Reuters correspondent, she is the Kathmandu representative of the Himalayan Trust, the organization set up by Hillary to support his various philanthropic ventures in the Sola Khumbu (these include the school at Khumjung, and two hospitals, one at Khunde and the other at Phaphlu). Elizabeth arranged for runners to handle all the mail that was sent to and from the expedition, and her help was indispensable. She was incidentally also a mine of information on what was going on in town, and on Himalayan expeditions generally.

We also negotiated with the American Embassy to send some scientific material back to the U.S. in their diplomatic pouch. But this arrangement turned out to be of limited value. The Embassy put tight restrictions on what could be sent this way, and in the event we trusted only one package of scientific data to this route. It arrived in San Diego several weeks after the ordinary mail looking as though it had been chewed by a dog.

Most of the remainder of the team arrived on August 3, and we prepared to leave on the 6th. John Evans and I went to a briefing with Mr. Sharma at the Ministry of Tourism on the day before we left. I felt a bit like a naughty schoolboy being summoned to the headmaster's office. He was very firm about adhering to our specified route, keeping radio schedules, and not starting on the route through the Khumbu icefall until September 1. This particular restriction rankled because it was so arbitrary, and the late date put us under considerable pressure to finish our complex scientific and climbing program before the weather turned bad. However, there was nothing we could do about it.

To ensure compliance two Nepalese liaison officers were assigned to the expedition. One, Yogendra Tapa, was in the police force, and became a popular member of the expedition. Not only was he personable with a flashing smile, but he was a strong climber. The other, Mingma Sherpa, was a doctor, one of only two sherpas ever to have earned a medical degree. He had obtained his training in India and, prior to the expedition, was the only doctor working in the small hospital in the village of Terhathum. We were impressed by his ability. He was a welcome asset to the expedition, and worked particularly with Lahiri on his experiments at Base Camp. Interestingly, he was the only sherpa who had the same uneven pattern of breathing during sleep that the westerners had. This was presumably due to the fact that he lived at a lower altitude. Possibly for the same reason he did not have the resilience to the rigors of high-altitude living that the other sherpas showed.

At last August 6 arrived, and it was a great relief to start moving toward our real objective and away from the administrative jungle of Kathmandu. Several of us had a last lunch at the Malla which, with beer, cost over $10— ridiculously expensive in this country, but justified as the last meal with table linen for three months. Then over to Mountain Travel where there was the usual chaos, but eventually the bus wheezed out of the compound. We drove east for two hours to the village of Dolalghat, and the road then wound north to the Tibetan border, 30 miles or so further on. We passed through some fine scenery though this was not easy to see through the bus windows which were both small and dirty.

One incident made a particular impression on me. Halfway through the trip a backpack fell off the top of the bus. It turned out to be Chris Pizzo's, and I was surprised at how strongly he reacted. In my dealings with him prior to the expedition he had always seemed very gentle, but now his drive and determination came out. I did not realize that this was a harbinger of things to come. As we reached Dolalghat a rainbow appeared over our first campsite, surely a good omen.

The three-week trek from Dolalghat to the Everest Base Camp has been described many times before, and there is little point in repeating it here. It is the classical trade route that has been used by countless merchants and

41

porters for centuries, and it is one of the most beautiful treks in the world. It was particularly interesting for me because I had covered exactly the same ground twenty years before. I even had a copy of my old diary with me, and found that the uphill climbs had lost none of their challenge. There is a beauty on the first day where the route goes solidly uphill for over 1,300 meters (4,000 feet). Unfortunately this was too much for Duane who had been laid low by flu a few days before. To his great disappointment he had to return to Kathmandu, and he eventually came in by helicopter with Karl Maret.

We had hoped that the trek would be a relaxing period with freedom from worry after the succession of crises in Kathmandu. However, it soon became clear that this was not to be. When we got up at 5 A.M. hoping to start on our way from Dolalghat, there was a severe shortage of porters. No local porters were available, and we only had the thirty-eight who had come out from Kathmandu. Various explanations were offered. Apparently work was available on the farmland at this time, and the prospect of carrying 30-kilogram (66-pound) loads through the torrential monsoon rains is unattractive, particularly as we were offering only the standard daily wage of about $2. This shortage of porters was to plague us all the way to Namche Bazar. At one stage one of the sherpas walking in with us who had very little time for the lowland porters came up with a novel plan. This was to promise to pay any porters who went all the way to Namche Bazar half pay for the return trip, and then renege on this agreement in three or four days' time when porters became more plentiful. I am glad to say that this rather dishonest plan fell through.

John Evans was reluctant to go ahead leaving the majority of the loads behind. We finally settled on a solution—Steve Boyer and Chris Kopczynski moved ahead with thirty-five porters and loads, and the rest of us sat around while Sonam Girme, our chief porter, went off in search of additional porters. He dispatched naiches, porter foremen who recruit porters for whom they are responsible.

The day was extremely hot with the tropical sun blazing down out of a cloudless sky. We were at an altitude of only 630 meters (2,000 feet), considerably lower than Kathmandu, and indeed the lowest point of our whole trek. We were camped by an enormous river, the Sun Kosi, and during the afternoon some of us took a swim. There was a terrific current, but it was the only way to keep cool. In the evening we walked into the nearby village, and were disconcerted to find several sections of the laboratory hut that had been abandoned. They had been sent with an advance group a few days before but the awkward panels were unpopular loads.

By evening additional porters had been found, and we set off by 6 A.M. the following morning, very relieved to be moving at last in the direction of

Everest. The two-week trek to Namche Bazar is a good hard walk that helps everybody get into shape for the rigors to come. Typically we rose at 5:30 and were off an hour later after tea and biscuits. This was often the best part of the day with clear, crisp mornings as we got higher, and I had plenty of opportunity to go over the science program again and again in my own mind and to discuss it with others. After four hours or so we would stop for lunch, usually by a stream. This was a substantial meal with omelets, potatoes, and tea, following which most of us lounged around for an hour or two washing clothes, reading, or just getting to know each other. Then on again in the afternoon for another two or three hours to reach our evening campsite by 4 or 5 P.M. The evening meal was usually followed by early bed in preparation for the next dawn's start.

There were many hours of just slogging uphill, but there were plenty of incidents along the way. After two days we were in leech country. These unpleasant creatures lie in wait on a moist leaf or rock, standing up on end and waving around when they sense an approaching victim. There is usually no sensation when they fasten themselves onto your skin, and the first indication is often a large red blood stain on a sock, which leads you to a fat, engorged black leech. Sometimes they are difficult to remove, and the bite often continues to bleed because they inject an anticlotting substance. In fact, this material was extracted from leeches, and used extensively in medicine in the last century to prevent coagulation.

The leeches are more of a nuisance than a danger, although we did have one sherpa who had a leech bite on his foot which developed into an ulcer and prevented him from climbing. They can certainly be very unpleasant. Mike Weis had one find its way on to his face while he was asleep in his tent during the night, and another dropped onto my neck from the ceiling when I was eating in one of the sherpa houses.

After two days we came across an Australian anthropologist and his wife who were living in the village of Risingo, studying ritual in the Thamangs, a local hill tribe. Jim Milledge and I went to visit them, and Jim, who has a photographic memory, astonished them by describing what houses were in the village twenty years ago when he walked in for the 1960–61 expedition.

By August 13 we had reached Those, one of the biggest villages on the trail. We walked across the precarious suspension bridge over the Khimti Khola River; the bridge was supported by enormous iron chains that had been forged in this village, which used to be a center for iron work. Generally you take your life in your hands on Nepalese bridges. A little further on they are festooned with Buddhist prayer flags presumably to increase their longevity, and it is said that the Nepalese repair them only when they break. Certainly there have been a number of hair-raising incidents involving expeditions; during the American 1963 expedition a bridge failed with a number of porters on it, and several floundered in the river, but fortunately nobody was killed. When the porters arrive at a particularly rickety example, they usually scamper across as fast as they can, one by one.

At Those we had another holdup because of difficulties with porters. We had just ensconced ourselves for the night in an empty schoolhouse that Mingma had found, when John Evans was called back to a ridge a couple of miles from Those. There the porters were having an angry confrontation with Sonam Girme, and refusing to continue with their loads. We never did get to the bottom of the story. However, it seems that the porters insisted on being paid then and there, and apparently Sonam Girme struck one of them who he thought was a troublemaker. To hit a man is an unforgivable breach of etiquette in this part of the world; defiant faces can be placed within half an inch of each other, but there is no jostling. Consequently Sonam was in great difficulties.

Mingma talked to the porters at length, finally convincing them to bring their loads into camp. How they found their way down the steep hill in the dark and across that crazy suspension bridge will always be a mystery to me. John Evans reported that he tried to look as formidable as possible while not understanding a word of what was going on. The upshot was that many of the porters abandoned the expedition at this point, and we had great trouble finding replacements. We suspected that Sonam Girme was persona non grata with the lowland porters.

By way of explanation it should be pointed out that there is a world of difference between the sherpas and the lowland porters, although both groups are inhabitants of Nepal. The sherpas are originally from Tibet, and rarely go down to the valleys; they are proud, intelligent, and ambitious. By contrast, the lowland porters (who are mainly Thamangs) generally live a menial laborer existence. Sonam, a wealthy, successful sherpa, probably had a very low opinion of the porters.

Jim Milledge and I agreed that these lowland porters were the only group in Nepal whose standard of living seemed not to have improved in the last twenty years. Most of them were still dressed in tattered loin cloths, and many were barefoot. Their pay was a miserable 24 rupees ($2) a day, from which they had to buy their own food. By contrast, a bottle of Nepalese beer cost 25 rupees, though admittedly this is exorbitant.

In Those we were visited by an old Nepalese woman whose twelve-year-old son was critically ill. He was seen by Mingma and Dave Graber who thought he probably had tuberculous meningitis, and was certainly dying. Apparently he had been misdiagnosed by a health worker in the village. This was a tragic error as a hospital with reasonable medical service is in Jiri only two hours away. The boy died soon after.

We ran medical clinics for the local population every evening; naturally there was no shortage of medical help though Frank Sarnquist, Peter Hackett, Dave Graber, Steve Boyer, and Mingma Sherpa did most of this work. As in any remote, undeveloped country, we saw many examples of advanced diseases that are now almost never seen in the U.S. Of course, the amount of good that can be done in one visit is limited, and some expedition doctors have claimed that these itinerant clinics are in fact harmful. I do not think this is so, particularly now that there are health clinics at intervals along the route, and patients can be referred to them. One area where we certainly did more good than harm was extracting teeth, which was Steve Boyer's specialty. We were sorry he was not with us in Risingo where we saw an old woman with a tooth abscess. The local blacksmith had pulled a tooth, but apparently it was the wrong one!

At Those we had to split up again because of the porter shortage. We were now beginning to get worried that we would be delayed beyond August 30 in establishing Base Camp. It was essential to start on the icefall route on September 1, the earliest date allowed by the Ministry of Tourism, because logistics were so complicated with our science objectives that we needed all available time before the winter closed in. We decided that an advance party consisting of Davey Jones, Chris Kopczynski, Glenn Porzak, Mike Weis, Dave Graber, Chris Pizzo, Frank Sarnquist, Brownie Schoene, Rick Peter, and Mingma Sherpa should move off with no porters (only a kitchen boy), and travel light and fast. The plan was to eat and spend nights in "tea houses" (Nepalese guest houses).

The advantages of this strategy were that this group could get to Namche to start acclimatizing, and also to begin moving the loads that were stored there to Base Camp. This left John Evans, Jim Milledge, Larry Lahiri, Bob Winslow, Mickey Samaja, Sonam Girme, and myself in Those with one or two kitchen staff. Rodney Korich and Steve Boyer were a little way behind with another 65 loads, and a final group was bringing up the rear with Sherpa Young Tensing. Jeff Lowe had been delayed in the U.S. by a family illness, and would catch up later.

By August 17 we reached Sete. It was teeming with rain, and we put up in a house near the gompa (Buddhist temple). Here we shared a large room with a Nepalese couple and their young child. During the evening there was a religious ceremony, apparently a baptism, in which a visiting priest recited a ritual text, and wafted incense smoke over the child. The child was very good and hardly made a sound even when it breathed the incense smoke.

However, it was odd to be awakened by its cry during the night, and also a bit strange to hear the noises of suckling.

In Sete we met a young American who was working in Namche for UNESCO and he told us a gruesome story about leeches. Some months previously a small leech had entered one of his nostrils when he was drinking from a mountain stream. The leech eventually grew to be 8 inches long with a sucker as big as a nickel and it caused considerable obstruction to his nose and nasopharynx— when it was removed (with great difficulty) they sent it to the Smithsonian museum! The effect of this cautionary tale was to increase everybody's respect for leeches considerably. Incidentally, we never drank directly from streams. Each of us had been issued a special filter cup through which drinking water was passed to purify it.

At about this time I discovered the wonders of the Sony Walkman cassette player. Several members of the expedition had these, but I had not brought one. However, when Rick Peters set off with the advance party he decided to travel as lightly as possible and he lent me his set. I was rapidly converted. At first sight it is bizarre to think of someone walking in a remote part of Nepal wearing a pair of earphones and listening to a Haydn Mass, but this was an ideal way of passing the time during an uneventful uphill slog. Sometimes the trail winds up a mountain for three or four hours and there is nothing much else you can do; the ground is so rocky that every step has to be watched, and I was too short of breath to talk. A Beethoven string quartet was ideal under these conditions. In the later stages of the expedition I was glad that my tentmate, Jim Milledge, had a Walkman with two pairs of earphones, and we spent many pleasant hours listening to music together deep inside our sleeping bags. When my wife, Penny, walked in to Base Camp near the end of the expedition, she brought a Walkman, which was a great success.

We passed through the charming European-like village of Junbesi, and started on the long pull up to the Trakshindu Pass where there was a fine Buddhist monastery. Since the rain was hosing down Mickey Samaja and I decided to pay it a visit. There was a fascinating gompa where I signed the guest book and made a small contribution. Large figures of Buddha arranged around the walls could just be discerned in the dim light. But the most interesting section was upstairs where we saw several monks squatting in a line, each holding an enormous sacred book on his knees. The pages were perhaps 6 inches by 3 feet in size, and the monks were systematically chanting their way through their own text. Each book was different, but the sounds, rather like a Gregorian chant, melded beautifully. We were told that the whole library of the monastery was read in this way every year. We saw monks of all ages, including a novice who was only six years old. As we left the monastery I was

46

astonished to meet a monk wearing a "UCLA Bruins" T-shirt. He spoke excellent English and it turned out that he had taught sherpa language at UCLA and Berkeley.

There was a long tough descent from Trakshindu to the village of Manidingma, the lowest point on the trek. The whole area was flooded, and there was no place to pitch tents. We stayed in a smelly cowshed, which became known as "cow shit cottage." It became something of a household name on the expedition. Whenever things got really tough we reminded each other of the night at Manidingma. The cows that had been occupying the room before we arrived naturally resented our invasion, and one came in to join us during the night. My diary notes that I had to get up at one stage during the night to shake fleas out of my pajama pants. We had good and bad campsites throughout the trek, but Manidingma was rock bottom.

The next day was a red-letter one because we reached the great Dudh Kosi River. Dudh means "milk," and the river derives its name from the milky appearance resulting from its tumultuous flow. As I stood mesmerized by the violence of the torrent I realized that some of the water came from Everest itself. Two days later we were walking up the beautiful valley of the Dudh Kosi through the charming village of Chaunrikharki when we were astonished first to hear, then see, a helicopter flying very high above the valley, in and out of the thick clouds. We realized that this must be carrying Duane Blume and Karl Maret together with the liquid nitrogen. After two weeks of plodding along for six or seven hours a day when the scientific aspects of the expedition seemed very far away, this was a reminder that there would soon be work to do. It was very enterprising of the Nepalese pilot to fly in during these unsettled monsoon conditions, and we later learned that he just found a window in the cloud for a landing at Thyangboche before all view of the ground disappeared.

We later learned that Duane and Karl's departure from Kathmandu had provoked some tension between them. Space and weight were at a premium on the helicopter, of course, and Duane had a number of essential supplies to bring in, with the liquid nitrogen being the prime payload. He was understandably miffed when Karl insisted on including his harp! I wish I could report that Karl was a competent harpist, and that he entertained us at Base Camp with lilting Gaelic songs after dinner. However, I only heard him tuning the thing on three or four occasions, and suspect that he is a beginner.

Sunday, August 23. Another red-letter day. We got off at 6 A.M. looking forward to arriving in Namche Bazar, the largest town of the Sola Khumbu, and the home of the sherpas. From here we would be on familiar ground all the way to Base Camp. As we wound our way up the steep hill to Namche we had our first spectacular view of Everest peeping over Nuptse. This fine view had to be a good omen, just as the rainbow that we saw over our first camp at Dolalghat as we arrived surely meant good fortune.

As we watched the clouds coming and going over the summit my mind went back to Mallory's description of Everest when the first reconnaissance expedition of 1921 had its first view of the mountain from Kampa Dzong in Eastern Tibet. "It was a perfect morning as we plodded up the barren slopes above our camp . . . we had mounted perhaps a thousand feet when we stayed and turned, and saw what we came to see. There was no mistaking the two great peaks in the west: that to the left must be Makalu, grey, severe, and yet distinctly graceful, and the other away to the right—who could doubt its identity? It was a prodigious white fang excrescent from the jaw of the world."[2]

I also recalled the other momentous event of that period in June 1921. The expedition had just buried the body of Dr. Kellas, an outstanding physiologist and climber, who had suddenly and unexpectedly died as they were crossing the pass at about 5,200 meters (17,200 feet). Kellas had worked with J. S. Haldane, one of the fathers of modern respiratory physiology, and it was a sobering thought that the first man to die on the first Everest expedition was a physiologist. Mallory felt the loss particularly keenly, and tried to name a mountain near Everest after Kellas, but the name never stuck. I sometimes wondered how we could give this pioneer physiologist and climber some recognition.

Namche looked much more attractive than I remembered it twenty years ago. A river runs down through the center and this is surrounded by gardens. Many houses have painted window frames and are set in serried rows—all against a background of green hills and blue sky. Most of the expedition were assembled here, and it was particularly good to be reunited with Duane and Karl. We visited Sonam Girme's beautiful home with his collection of sacred books, and photos of old expeditions. His wife welcomed us very graciously. After lunch I walked up to the police post with Mingma to inquire about using their radio in an emergency. However, this was clearly forbidden and, furthermore, we were asked a lot of awkward, unanswerable questions about passport numbers, etc. The moral was to avoid the police in this part of the world as far as possible.

Next morning I walked up to the village of Khunde to visit the Hillary hospital there. I was alone, and I followed a group of schoolchildren including a few giggling adolescent girls up the steep path over the ridge above Namche. Little wonder that the sherpas carry so well at high altitude if they climb 300 meters (1,000 feet) or so every morning for school. The children were on their way to the school in Khumjung that Hillary built at the end of our expedition in 1961. I took a left turn before we reached the village, and thought that I had lost my way for a while, but suddenly there was a chorten with prayer flags, and then the beautiful village of Khunde laid out in front.

Reaching the hospital, I asked a cleaning woman for the doctor and was directed to a door marked "Surgery." I knocked briefly and walked in only to find Dr. John Reekie, the resident doctor from New Zealand, in the middle of pulling a tooth from a very nervous old sherpani patient. Fortunately he was not put off his stroke and managed to get out one grotty old molar, although he decided not to persevere with the next. His wife, Sue, was acting as his assistant; she was a pretty New Zealand girl dressed as a sherpani, and she gave me some excellent homemade shortbread. John told me of his plans to go to England for some pediatric training, and I hope I gave him some good advice.

At Namche we were able to pay off the lowland porters, and move most of the loads onto yaks. In spite of their enormous size, these fine animals can move agilely up the moraine of the glacier all the way to Base Camp. They are owned by yak herders who are generally splended looking Tibetans with turquoise earrings, high leather boots, and plaited hair tied on top of their heads. The yaks have a will of their own and occasionally show it by rolling on the loads, so we did not entrust the delicate scientific equipment to them. They can also be stubborn. One that had been given a gigantic load in Sonam Girme's yard responded by lying down and refusing to get up. Sonam's reply to this gambit was to pick up a generous handful of yak dung and ram it down the miserable animal's throat. This indignity was sufficient to get the yak moving smartly.

In the afternoon we left for Thyangboche, a famous Buddhist monastery on a magnificent site. The trail to Thyangboche winds down a hill to the Imja Khola River, and this is followed by a long haul up to the monastery. As I puffed up this I remembered that someone had sent a pony for John Hunt to ride up the hill in 1953, and I regretted my lack of influence.

Just before I reached the river I met an old sherpa man who looked faintly familiar, but before we could get into conversation a group of yaks came along the narrow trail, and I had to move out of their way. Larry Lahiri was coming along behind, and he recognized the sherpa as Khunjo Chumbi of yeti fame. He was the village elder of Khumjung who was entrusted to safeguard the yeti's scalp when it was taken by Hillary around the world in 1960. The yeti, or abominable snowman, has always been newsworthy, particularly since 1951 when Shipton and Ward photographed some tracks that looked as though they were made by a giant biped. There was a good deal of excitement when the village of Khumjung produced a scalp that they said came from a yeti. Chumbi had a fantastic trip; he visited Chicago, Paris, and London where he was received at Buckingham Palace. The yeti scalp was subsequently identified as the skin of a blue bear, but Chumbi must have dined out on his experiences for a very long time indeed.

Every expedition to Everest through Nepal passes Thyangboche, and everyone agrees it is the high point of the trek to Base Camp. "My senses were intoxicated by the fantastic surroundings; Thyangboche must be one of the most beautiful places in the world," wrote Hunt, a man not normally given to superlatives. The monastery is ringed by magnificent Himalayan peaks, and in the distance is Everest itself with its characteristic snow plume rearing up behind the great wall of Nuptse. We arrived in rain but the following morning I was awakened at 5 A.M. by loud gongs from the gompa—an impressive and slightly threatening sound—followed by horns—very low notes with warbling semi and quarter tones. While the monks were chanting I walked outside and, as the morning mists cleared, Everest and its magnificent companions came into view.

After breakfast those of us who had just arrived in Thyangboche had an audience with the High Lama. He is an impressive man with a fine face, handsome robe, and dignified manner. He has seen all the Everest expeditions trek past Thyangboche since Nepal was opened to foreigners in the late 1940s. Charles Houston visited him in 1950 when he was a 14-year-old boy and had only recently been selected as the reincarnate lama. We filed into his U-shaped room where there were the usual anachronisms of Nepal. On the floor was an elegant Tibetan rug, but around the walls were hung various posters showing the flags of the world, and a certificate from the Chattanooga Rotary Club in Tennessee.

We had a long, interesting conversation with Mingma acting as an interpreter. We asked the lama about mountain sickness because the monastery is at an elevation of 3,900 meters (12,700 feet), and the monks used to move freely between there and the Rongbuk monastery across the range on the Tibetan side. The lama said that the monks had been aware of mountain sickness for a very long time, and attributed it to the special winds of high places. Interestingly, this is the explanation that José deAcosta offered when he gave the first clear description of mountain sickness almost 400 years ago. I was hoping that the lama would give us a reference to early views on mountain sickness in one of the Buddhist texts, but was disappointed. This would have been something of a coup in the history of respiratory physiology.

Because of his long experience with Everest expeditions we asked him what was the most important ingredient for success. I expected a deep spiritual

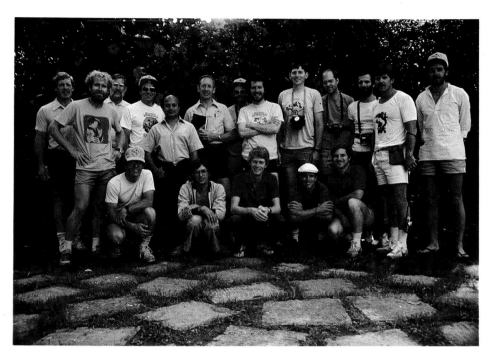

Members of the expedition at Kathmandu prior to the trek in. Back row (L. to R.): Evans, Boyer, Blume, Kopczynski, Lahiri, West, Jones, Hackett, Graber, Winslow, Samaja, Schoene, Pizzo. Front row: Sarnquist, Korich, Peters, Weis, Porzak. Absent: Lowe, Maret, Milledge. (*John P. Evans*)

First camp during trek at Dolalghat. (*Christopher J. Pizzo*)

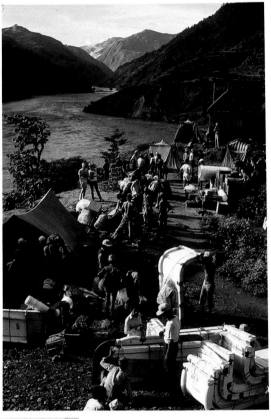

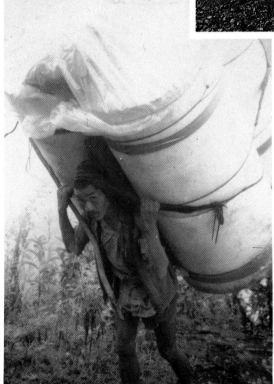

Lowland porter carrying a load of insulating material. (*John P. Evans*)

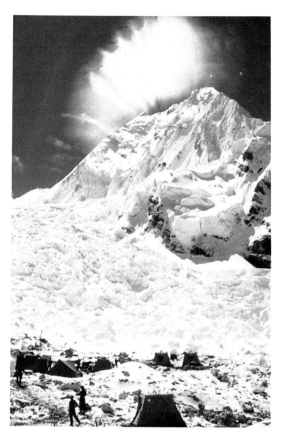

Base Camp with Nuptse on the right. (*Christopher J. Pizzo*)

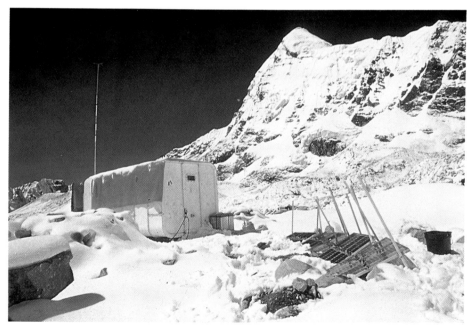

Base Camp laboratory (5,400 meters; 17,700 feet). (*Sukhamay Lahiri*)

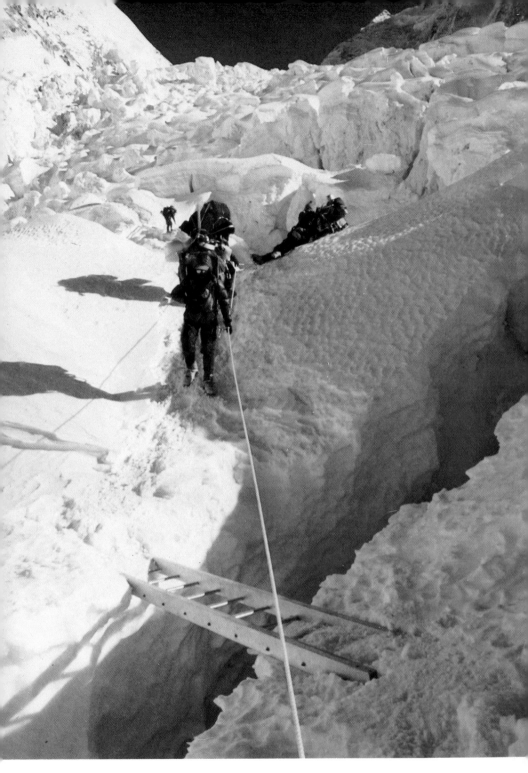

Large crevasse in Khumbu icefall.   (*Karl H. Maret*)

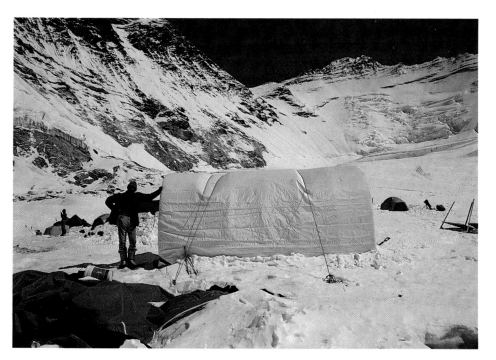

Main laboratory at Camp 2 (6,300 meters; 20,700 feet). *(John B. West)*

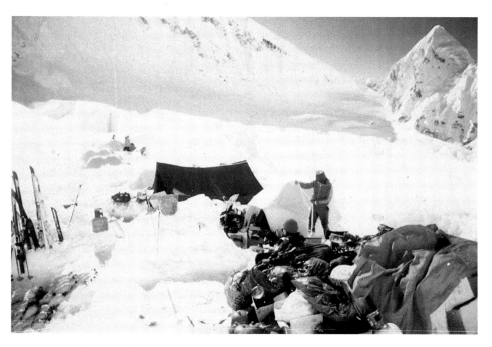

Camp 1 (5,950 meters; 19,500 feet). *(David J. Graber)*

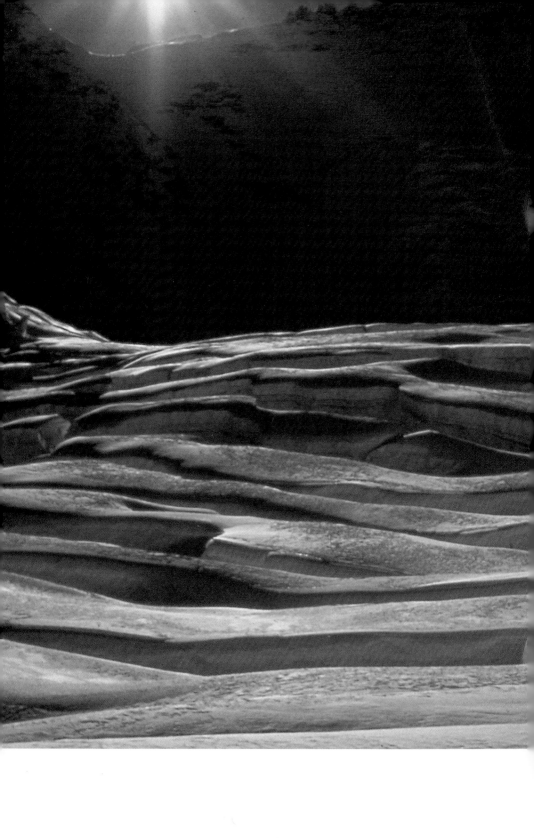

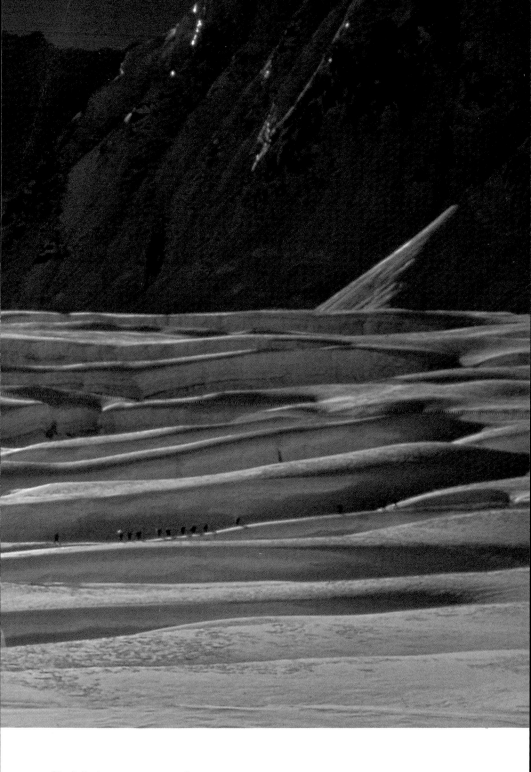

Undulating snow near the top of the icefall.   (*Robert M. Winslow*)

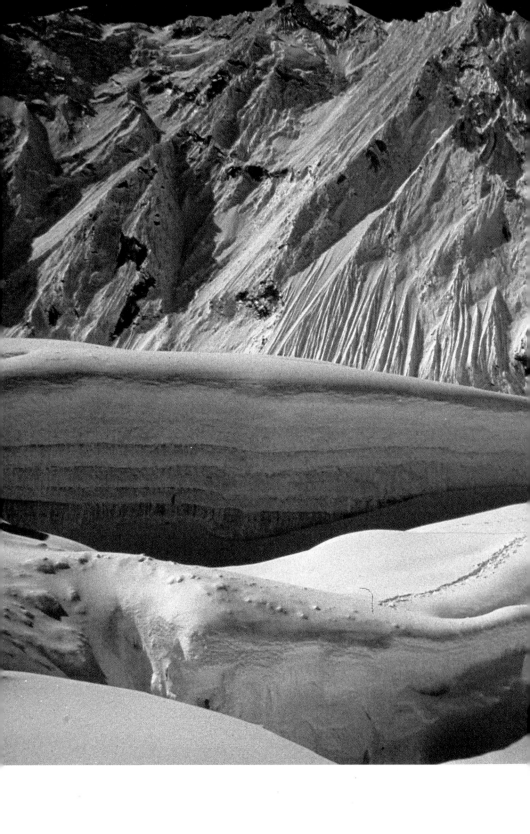

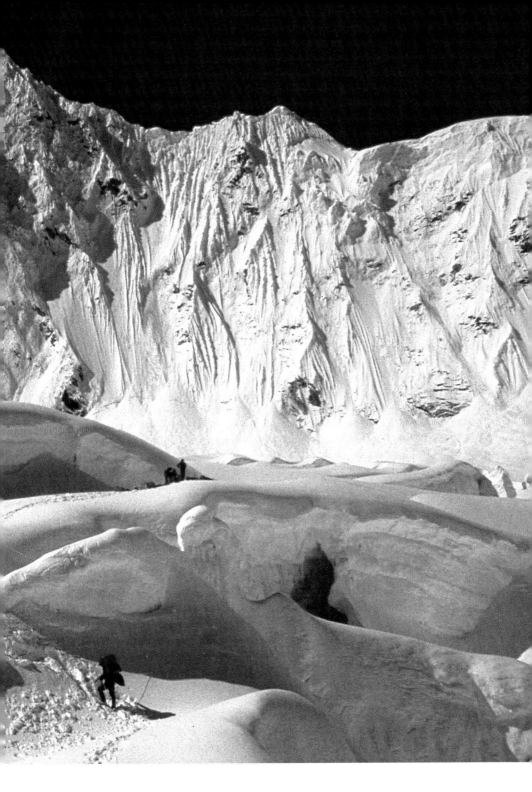

Nearing Camp 1; Nuptse in the background.   (*Robert B. Schoene*)

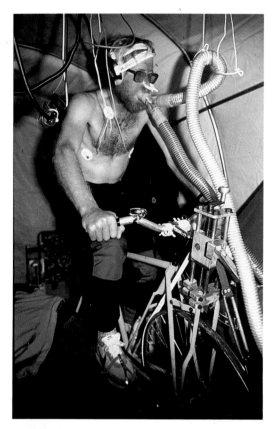

Steve Boyer on the stationary bicycle in the Camp 2 laboratory. (*Karl H. Maret*)

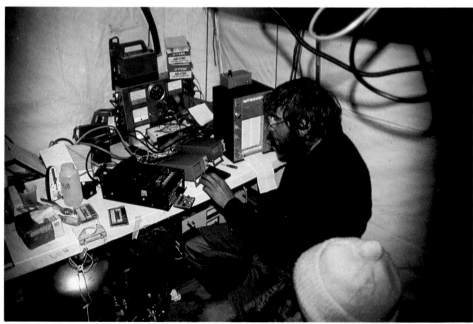

Karl Maret checking equipment in the Camp 2 laboratory.   (*Robert M. Winslow*)

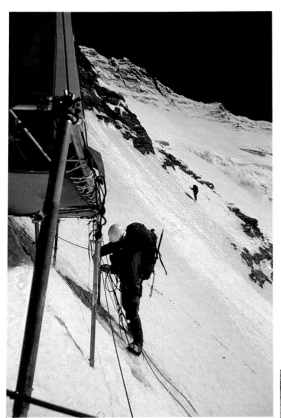

Camp 3 (7,250 meters; 23,800 feet). (*David J. Graber*)

View down into the Western Cwm from near Camp 3. Camp 2 can be seen as a tiny dot. (*Christopher J. Pizzo*)

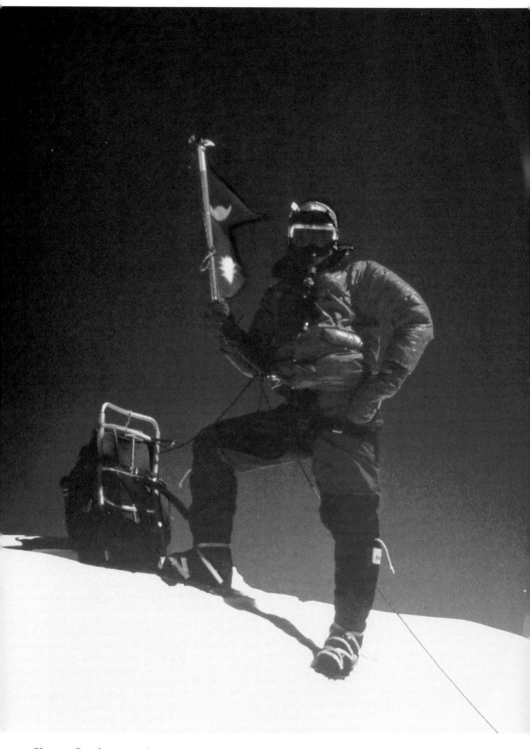

Sherpa Sondare on the summit (8,848 meters; 29,028 feet).   (*Chris Kopczynski*)

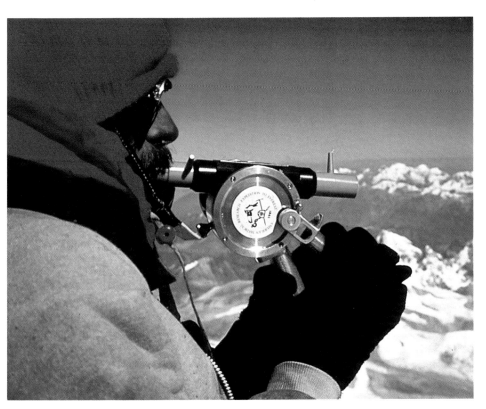

Chris Pizzo on the summit taking samples of air from his lungs.
(*Sherpa Young Tenzing*)

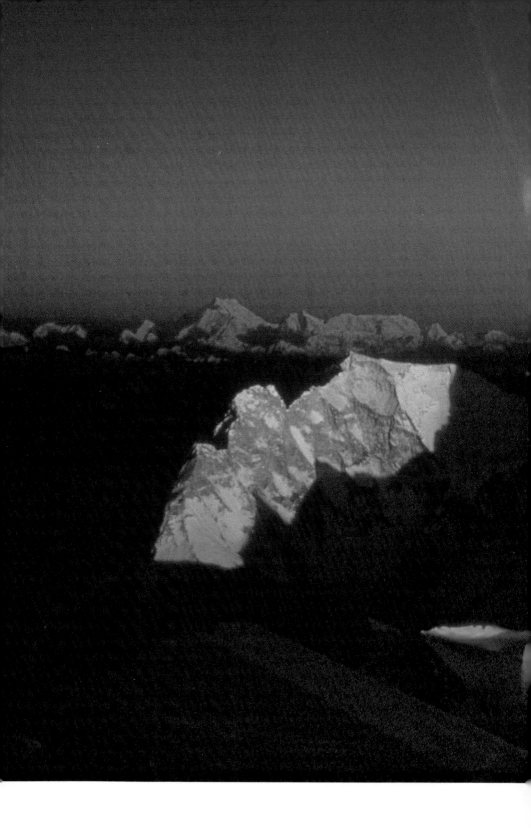

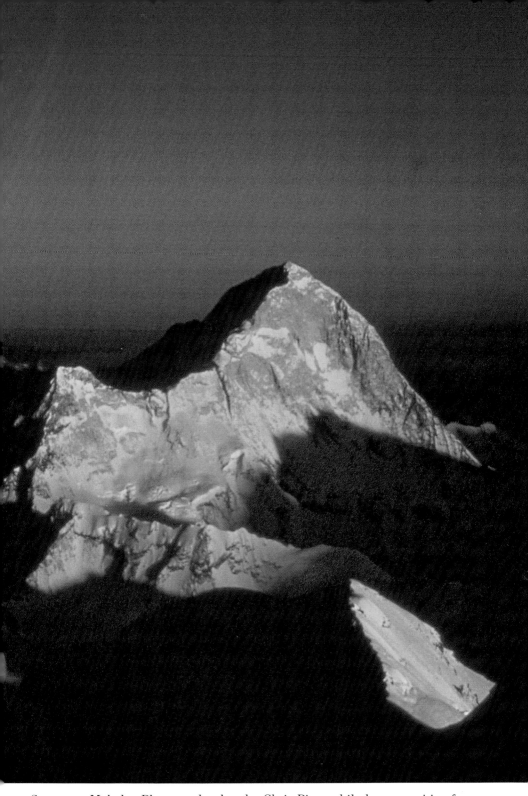

Sunset on Makalu. Photograph taken by Chris Pizzo while he was waiting for Peter Hackett. (*Christopher J. Pizzo*)

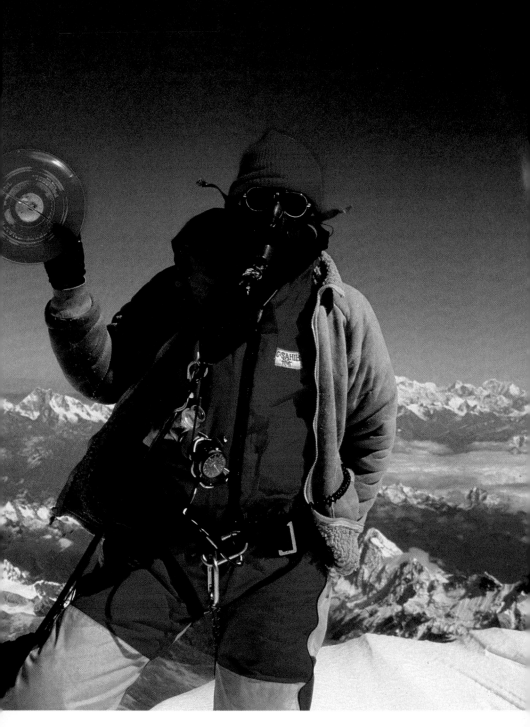

Pizzo about to make the high-altitude Frisbee record. (*Sherpa Young Tenzing*)

Buddhist reply, but instead his answer was luck! As it turned out, he was absolutely right. To be fair, he did go on to add that good personal relationships among the expedition participants were vital, and that we should also be charitable in our dealings with others.

Next day we set off on the trail to Pheriche, through a beautiful forest of rhododendrons. Though they were not in bloom we could imagine the visual effect of these acres of large flowers. I was with Jim Milledge and Larry Lahiri, and we spent some time looking for the house of Dawa Tenzing who was the sirdar on our 1960–61 expedition and who was with General Bruce on the 1924 Everest expedition. It was moving to think about this link with one of the earliest and most famous of the Everest expeditions, the one on which Mallory and Irving disappeared. We were unable to find Dawa Tenzing's house in spite of directions given to us by an old woman who gesticulated from an upstairs window in what was presumably the nunnery at Deboche. It was a pity; apparently Dawa Tenzing can recall the events of 1924 quite clearly.

Dominating the skyline to our right was the magnificent peak of Ama Dablam, a fang of a mountain if there ever was one. This had special memories for the three of us who had been on the 1960–61 expedition because we spent the winter not far from the base of the mountain. During that time four members of the expedition, Barry Bishop, Mike Gill, Wally Romanes, and Mike Ward, made the first ascent via the spectacular south ridge. It was a magnificent climb on a route with great technical difficulty and much exposure, but it was an unauthorized ascent and got the expedition into a good deal of hot water. It took all of Hillary's tact and diplomacy to smooth that one over.

We arrived at Pheriche in time for lunch in the building of the Himalayan Rescue Association. This clinic was started by a Japanese surgeon from Tokyo, and is staffed part of the year by Peter Hackett, so we were given a warm welcome. The clinic was set up because trekkers heading for the Everest Base Camp pass through Pheriche, and acute mountain sickness is common.

Mountain sickness is a constellation of complaints including headache, fatigue, dizziness, palpitations, insomnia, loss of appetite, nausea, and sometimes vomiting. It occurs in trekkers or climbers who ascend too rapidly for the normal processes of acclimatization to occur. There are striking differences between individuals, and some people can never acclimatize to the altitude at Pheriche, which is 4,240 meters (almost 14,000 feet). Most of our expedition had so far had little trouble with the altitude because we had been ascending gradually for three weeks. This is by far the best way to develop proper acclimatization, and is one of the reasons why expeditions like to walk in the whole way from Kathmandu. Some trekkers use acetazolamide (Diamox) to assist in acclimatization; there is evidence that this drug hastens the acclimatization process if the trekker has too little time to move up slowly enough, but the drug has a number of side effects and should be used cautiously.

Peter told us that acute mountain sickness had been extremely common here a few years ago. (The condition particularly affects young people for reasons that are not understood.) However, the incidence of mountain sickness has been enormously reduced by emphasizing the importance of gradual ascent, and the Himalayan Rescue Association can take a lot of the credit for this.

Occasionally trekkers develop one of the complications of acute mountain sickness, pulmonary edema (fluid in the lungs) or cerebral edema (fluid in the brain). The first is not particularly rare; in fact, we had three people associated with the expedition who developed this. The patient becomes very short of breath, especially on lying down at night, and the lips become blue indicating insufficient oxygen in the blood. If you put a stethoscope on the chest you can hear crackling sounds caused by fluid in the lung airways. The treatment is to get the subject down as quickly as possible and give him oxygen if it is available.

Cerebral edema is a much more ominous condition. The victim becomes confused, disoriented, and may even lose consciousness. Again the best treatment is to move him to a lower altitude. There have been a number of deaths from both pulmonary and cerebral edema near Pheriche over the years, but with wider appreciation of the importance of ascending slowly, these conditions are now much less common.

Although none of our expedition members specifically complained of mountain sickness, there was nevertheless a good deal of minor illness at this time. Jim Milledge had developed a severe cold in Namche that put him in bed for a few days. Both Dave Graber and Mike Weis had bouts of diarrhea. Duane Blume and Karl Maret were feeling the effects of altitude a bit, but this was to be expected since they had flown in to Namche by helicopter instead of sharing our gradual ascent.

Generally speaking, our expedition did not have a lot of trouble with gastrointestinal illness. Much of the credit for this goes to Frank Sarnquist who was adamant that the sherpas be scrupulous about hygiene; Frank gave them frequent lectures on the importance of handwashing before meals. Additionally, we brought in an enormous water-purifying system consisting of a filter and pump, which we lugged all the way up to Base Camp. Also each member had his own water filter based on a design from the NASA space program in case he needed to drink from a stream along the way. In general, though, this was discouraged. Some members took tablets of doxycycline as a prophylactic and this seemed to help (see Appendix D).

We were now within two days of Base Camp, and there was an air of expectation as we were poised to finish the last stages of the long trek. On August 28 Glenn Porzak, Chris Kopczynski, Steve Boyer, and Chris Pizzo worked on the route to Base Camp from Gorak Shep. This was on the moraine (rock debris) covering the Khumbu Glacier, and a way had to be found over several glacier streams. We had a glorious walk up the valley to Lobuya where most of us began to feel at least some effects of altitude. In fact, I arrived to find John Evans and Rick Peters about to head back to Pheriche because of headaches. We played some bridge in the afternoon and noted that Davey Jones's psychic no-trump bids (often successful) seemed more irritating to me than usual—no doubt the altitude.

I slept poorly that night, and woke up several times feeling suffocated. This is a common complaint, probably due to the periodic or "Cheyne-Stokes" breathing that everybody gets at high altitudes. The breathing waxes and wanes rhythmically; several deep sighing breaths are followed by several very shallow breaths, or even several seconds of no breathing at all—rather alarming at first if you are sharing a tent with someone who is doing it. All of us developed this condition during sleep at Base Camp and higher, though most of the sherpas did not. Their breathing remained steady during sleep. This was one of the topics that Larry Lahiri studied, and was related to the nervous factors controlling breathing at high altitudes.

During the evening meal Sonam Girme arrived having walked all the way from Namche in one day, a distance that took us three days. He appeared to be tense and under a lot of strain. This was partly because we were still uncertain about the whereabouts of the last group of loads being carried in by sherpa Sungdare. On August 29 Base Camp was sited by Porzak, Kopczynski, Boyer, Pizzo, and Sonam, though they retired down the glacier to Gorak Shep for the night.

Sunday, August 30, my diary takes up the story. "Fantastic day. Left Lobuya at 7:30 A.M. for Base Camp. Glorious walk to Gorak Shep, which took about two hours—tantalizing peeps of Nuptse, Pumori, Lindgren. Initially walked in a T-shirt and even wished I had shorts. Warm, slightly misty morning. Above Gorak Shep it got colder, and later it snowed. Fairly hard walk over the moraine—past fantastic ice pinnacles. Tremendously exhilarating to arrive at Base Camp at last. Had about 10 cups of tea when I arrived at about 12:30 P.M. (missed lunch). Then set to work to put up the Weatherport [the semirigid laboratory hut] on a flat area prepared by the sherpas. Distant sound of avalanches, and the icefall is dead ahead a few hundred yards away—this is it! Jim and I apparently have the Weatherport to ourselves tonight. I walked up with one of the yak herders—it is not easy to find your way over the moraine, which is poorly marked with cairns. Many yaks going up and down—very colorful. There are now eight sahibs in Base Camp—Davey Jones, Glenn Porzak, Chris Kopczynski, Chris Pizzo, Jim Milledge, Brownie Schoene, Steve Boyer, and myself."

So far so good. We are nicely on schedule for starting on the icefall route on September 1. The next two months will show whether the years of preparation have been worth it.

5

BASE CAMP, ICEFALL, AND ABOVE

"Drive through regardless"[1]

Base Camp is a bleak place to live in, but you have to give full marks for its view. The Khumbu Glacier is covered with rock debris, the boulders being anywhere from one to six feet in diameter. Before a tent can be pitched, a relatively flat platform has to be constructed by arranging small rocks. Naturally the resulting surface is hard and bumpy, though a sheet of plastic foam does wonders for sleep.

The most obvious and ominous feature of the scenery is the Khumbu ice-fall, which is directly behind. Some 600 meters (2,000 feet) high, and jammed with enormous ice blocks contorted into grotesque shapes, it seems to warn the newcomer that the Cooks Tour stops at Base Camp. On the left of the ice-fall is the enormous mass of the west shoulder of Everest itself leading down to a low point known as the Lho La on its left. Every now and then an avalanche thunders off this. Further to the left is the high col over which Mallory peered in 1921 when the first glimpse of the Khumbu icefall by a westerner was obtained. Still further to the left is Pumori, a magnificent conical peak that not only dominates the view to the west from Base Camp but is a prominent feature in any photograph taken looking west from the Western Cwm. To the right of the icefall is the west ridge of Nuptse, and its fluted north wall striding up to flank the southern part of the Western Cwm can be seen. The whole gallery of mountains makes man look very puny indeed.

As soon as Base Camp was established we set to work to erect the two laboratories. For the Base Camp we had chosen the Hansen Weatherport, a commercially available semirigid structure that had been used with great success during the construction of the Alaska pipeline. It consists of an aluminum frame over which are placed fiberglass blankets to give thermal insulation. There is a zipper door at one end, and a large plastic window at the other. The whole thing can be put together in a couple of hours, and Jim and I did just that the afternoon we arrived at Base Camp.

Rick Peters had constructed a plywood floor for the Weatherport when we were in Kathmandu. This exercise proved to be a good introduction to the frustrations of Nepal because the electrical supply to run the saw was off more than it was on. However, Rick beat that one as he did every other problem along the way with his inexhaustible drive and resourcefulness. (Incidentally, although we used the Weatherport primarily as a laboratory, it would make a very comfortable meeting or mess tent for any expedition, and we later sold it along with other equipment to the Canadians who were going to attempt Everest in the fall of the following year.)

For Camp 2 where conditions were expected to be much more rigorous, we designed the rigid hut made of plastic foam panels covered with Kevlar. This was essentially a scaled-down version of the Silver Hut of the 1960–61 expedition, but using more modern techniques. A big difference was that whereas we originally used the Silver Hut for sleeping and eating accommodation as well as a laboratory, this time the sleeping and eating would be done elsewhere so the hut could be much smaller and lighter. We were anxious to erect the hut at Base Camp, and test all the equipment in it, even though this would mean disassembling it to carry it to Camp 2. It seemed important to determine that everything worked properly in the relative comfort of Base Camp, rather than have some unpleasant surprise when everything was unpacked up in the remote Western Cwm.

The first job for the erection of both laboratories was to prepare a flat area on the glacier, which is covered by great heaps of stones that have to be rearranged to provide some sort of platform. Since the glacier is always slowly moving, platforms have a tendency to change their shape over the weeks. We were very relieved to find that assembling both laboratory structures was easy, and they were obviously going to function well. A minor disappointment was that water leaked through the ceiling of the rigid hut through junctions between the flanges of the panels when the sun thawed the snow. But this problem was easily solved by placing a plastic tarpaulin over the hut.

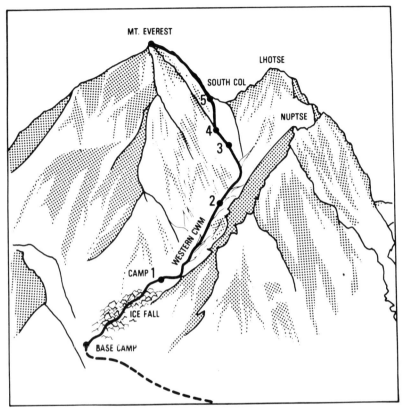

Figure 1.   View of Everest from the southeast showing the locations of the camps. The main laboratory was at Camp 2, altitude 6,300 meters (20,700 feet), and there was another laboratory at Base Camp (5,400 meters, 17,700 feet). (Compare Figure 2, page 74.)

A priority for testing the scientific equipment was to generate power, and Karl Maret had spent a great deal of time planning the generators and batteries. We were a little surprised to find that in this day and age lead-acid batteries are still the best bet in spite of their weight. The people at Gould Incorporated, a giant battery corporation, gave us a lot of help on this, and recommended marine-type batteries. The great advantage of these deep discharge batteries is that they continue to provide a satisfactory voltage even when their charge has been almost fully depleted. This was an important design feature for the expedition because we would be doing experiments during the night, and we hoped it would not be necessary to run the noisy generators at that time. We had shipped Teflon bottles of concentrated sulfuric acid from La Jolla in special custom-made boxes and I was surprised that the shipping people did not create more difficulties about this hazardous cargo. At Base Camp Jim Milledge and I diluted the concentrated acid for the batteries with clean snow checking the specific gravity with a hydrometer.

Karl had elected to make his own generators from Stihl chain-saw motors coupled to automobile alternators. There was an elaborate power control panel which allowed us to adjust the load on the alternators, and also to accept power at the same time from solar panels in the circuit. These panels were the most innovative feature of the system. After a long search, Karl persuaded the Matsushita Corporation of Tokyo (Panasonic) to lend us ten solar panels for converting sunlight into electricity. These are so expensive that the expedition could not hope to buy them.

These panels turned out to be a great success. They put out a total of 30 amps at some 15–18 volts, which was very nice "free power" indeed. The panels like intense solar radiation, and there was no shortage of that now that half of the atmosphere was below us. The panels also work best when they are kept cold and, of course, that too was no problem. We packed snow behind them so that they were oriented at right angles to the noon sun.

We also tested our two Hewlett Packard ear oximeters. This device measures the oxygen concentration in the blood from its color by using a light beam shining through the ear. Almost all the electronic equipment worked well in spite of its long and eventful trip from California. I was particularly anxious to get our ham radio working so that we could start daily radio schedules to Kathmandu. The Ministry of Tourism required daily reports of the progress of the expedition, and we could also order spares for equipment by getting messages to Mountain Travel.

While the scientists were setting up the laboratories, the climbers were coming to grips with their first major obstacle, the Khumbu icefall. The Everest Base Camp is dominated by the icefall, both physically and, one might say, spiritually. Ever since climbers have been attempting Everest from the south, the icefall has been a major challenge. When Mallory first saw it during the Everest reconnaissance of 1921, he wrote, "We reach the Col at 5:00 A.M., a fantastically beautiful scene . . . we have seen this western glacier [icefall] and are not sorry we have not to go up it. It is terribly steep and broken." Then in 1950, shortly after Nepal was opened to foreigners, the icefall was first seen at fairly close quarters by Dr. Charles Houston and H. W. Tilman. They too formed a very pessimistic view of it.

The following year a key reconnaissance was carried out by a party led by Shipton, and including Hillary and Ward, and they concluded that the icefall was climbable, though desperately unsafe. Hillary described his reactions in *High Adventure:* "Shipton was far from happy about subjecting sherpas to such a route—it hardly worked in with the deep-seated British tradition of respon-sibility and fair play. But, in my heart, I knew the only way to attempt this mountain was to modify the old standards of safety and justifiable risk and to meet the dangers as they came; to drive through regardless. Care and caution would never make a route through the icefall."

The Khumbu icefall is a frozen waterfall of ice formed as the glacier emerges from the Western Cwm and tumbles down the steep 600-meter (2,000-foot) slope to the lower part of the glacier where Base Camp is located. It is relatively narrow, squeezed between the west shoulder of Everest to the north and the giant wall of Nuptse to the south. The danger lies in its instability; enormous blocks of ice (seracs) as big as the room of a house assume crazy attitudes, and topple over from time to time. Since the route must go under these ice towers, it is a matter of Russian roulette whether an expedition member happens to be under one at the time it collapses.

All of us had had plenty of reminders of the dangers of the icefall. Several expedition members had known Jake Breitenbach, the young climber of the 1963 American expedition who was buried by one of these seracs early in their icefall reconnaissance. Our Base Camp cook, Ang Pema, had been on the same rope, and his misshapen nose broken at the time was a constant reminder of his accident. On our way from Lobuya to Gorak Shep we had passed the six cairns of stones erected by the Japanese expedition of 1970 to commemorate the sherpas who were buried in the icefall at that time. As I write this I am reminded of the three sherpas and climber who were killed in the icefall during the Canadian Everest expedition that took place just one year after ours. They were in the same place at almost the same time a year later. There but for the grace of God. . . .

I had my own phobia about the icefall; in the years of preparation for the expedition it often forced itself into my consciousness in the middle of the night. This phobia was not helped when we all had to fill in our "disaster plan" form that indicated how your body should be disposed of if the worst occurred. Some members were distinctly offhand about this—"throw it into the nearest crevasse" appeared several times.

When John Evans first saw the icefall about midday on August 31 his immediate impression was that it did not look as dangerous as in 1971. This view was confirmed by Steve Boyer who climbed high on the moraine behind Base Camp during the afternoon, and brought back Polaroid photos that sug-gested that, by keeping to the left, a route might be found up it without too much difficulty. But the following day would tell.

Kop, Chris, Steve, and Glenn were up at 4:00 A.M. on September 1, and by 5 they were heading for the icefall. They found the going best on the left side, and were jubilant when they came down, reporting that they had fixed some 360 meters (1,200 feet) of rope by 10:00 A.M. They believed that they had climbed two-thirds of the way to the top. On the following morning Steve and Chris went as high as they could, extending the route while John and Kop improved the route lower down. This party came back a little less optimistic because although they had pushed the route a good deal further, they were still not into the Cwm.

However, the next day Steve and Kop reached a point that they considered suitable for siting Camp 1, while Brownie and Glenn continued work on the lower end of the route. Another 2,000 feet of rope were fixed on the following day, though Brownie reported that one part of the route was very unpleasant with large seracs and crevasses. There was a good deal of elation at this stage because of the rapid progress. Finding a route through the icefall can sometimes take as long as two weeks, and some expeditions have found their way barred by an enormous crevasse, necessitating a halt while special ladders are brought in.

At this point we had something of a setback. The weather deteriorated, and snow fell steadily during the 5th, 6th, and 7th. Avalanche dangers in the icefall made it too dangerous for work, and the climbers took a well-earned rest. On September 5, a slide from the west shoulder of Everest nearly reached the icefall route, giving Steve who was working on the lower portion a scare. This raised the question of whether the route should be moved to the right away from the west shoulder.

Then two days later I was working in the laboratory hut when a group of sherpas rushed in. Initially I thought it was an abrupt retreat during a snowball fight, but when I looked out of the door I could see a lot of spindrift coming down off Everest, and there was a high wind. Many of the sherpas were tearing off down the moraine. This was my first introduction to the wind blast that heralds an avalanche, and a chill went down my spine. The following day the same thing happened at about 8:00 P.M. while we were in the mess tent. I ran outside and soon regretted it. A great wind with fine snow bore down, quickly covering me from head to foot.

But the most dramatic event occurred early the following night. My diary recounts it: "I went to sleep early but at 9:30 P.M. was awakened by Jim who shouted at me to hold the tent down. Enormous avalanche with a gale of wind which caught our Hillary tent from behind. We both held it down as best we could. Wind continued for ages—I was scared stiff. Lots of shouting from the rest of the camp. After it was over I could not get to sleep. Partly just scared. Partly dwelling on how foolish it would be to be killed in this remote area . . . ."

Several tents were blown over by the wind blast, and the following day

Sonam recommended that we move the whole camp about 100 yards east out of the avalanche path. Most of the tents were moved, but we left the two laboratories and a stone hut where they were. This last was made with walls of piled-up rocks with a tarpaulin as roof, and its construction had consumed several days. It was originally built to be a mess hut, but we converted it into a storage area, and built another stone mess hut in a safer area.

Up until this time no sherpas had been in the icefall; all the work had been done by sahibs. On September 7 we had a Puja, a religious ceremony, to offer gifts to the mountain gods and pray for safety during the expedition. In retrospect this was certainly one of the high points of the early part of the expedition.

First the sherpas set up a stone altar on which they placed food and drink. The expedition's offering was a bottle of Ballantyne's scotch whiskey and another of California Cabernet Sauvignon. Next a long line of Buddhist prayer flags perhaps 100 meters long was strung across the glacier below the icefall. These flags remained in place throughout the whole expedition. Then the ceremony started.

Two sherpas who had trained as priests intoned prayers from sacred texts. These were small versions of the kind of books I had seen in the monastery at Trakshindu—the pages were long and narrow with the hinge at the top. From time to time during the chanting, the priests and the rest of us who were standing around threw small amounts of sacred rice into the air. All the sherpas and sahibs were appropriately solemn, though there was a good deal of photography.

After a long period of this, the food offerings were passed around. Then Sonam Girme dispensed the whiskey in the bottle cap—each member and sherpa had two swigs, and it tasted pretty potent at that altitude—and the wine was poured into cupped hands. The whole ceremony was a delightful mixture of formal ritual and local expediency and lasted about an hour. This Buddhist ceremony clearly had interesting parallels with those of other religions.

After the Puja the sherpas were willing to work in the icefall, though nobody ever lost his respect for it. One day coming down through it I met a group of sherpas climbing up with their loads. Several were mumbling "Om mani padme hum" (Greeting, thou jewel of the lotus), the traditional Buddhist prayer, indicating that the sherpas were just as apprehensive about the icefall as I was.

John Evans gave a short talk about the nature of the expedition, and introduced the members. Then the sherpas were invited to come forward one by one to be introduced and give their name, village, age, and number of previous expeditions. Some of the sherpas claimed to be much older than they looked, and Peter explained that many have little idea of their true age. Also several of the sherpas, especially the younger ones, seemed to have been on an astonishingly large number of expeditions, but we all applauded appropriately.

Following this I spoke briefly about the science program, and Davey Jones demonstrated what a climber would look like wearing all the summit scientific equipment. We invited interested sherpas for a tour of the laboratory, and the young ones particularly had their eyes out on stalks. The younger sherpas were generally fascinated by the scientific aspects of the expedition, and frequently came into the laboratory to watch some of the experiments (though it must be admitted that in the later stages of the expedition at Camp 2 this was the only warm place in camp).

The Puja and the subsequent meeting with the sherpas were enormously successful, and I think marked the beginning of the close relationship that had to exist among everybody if the mountain was going to be climbed. We had our differences with the sherpas from time to time but, in general, no one could wish for a better group of people to work with. They are cheerful, good-humored, and loyal; indeed, many veteran Himalayan climbers have argued that one of the best parts of climbing Mt. Everest is working with the sherpas. We had had an example of their humor a few days earlier. As part of the required clothing issue, we gave them some German army surplus jackets. In response to this they all dressed up in these to have their photograph taken along with a large sign saying American Medical Research Expedition to Everest!

During these days when the weather precluded work in the icefall, we had several afternoon science seminars in the mess hut. These consisted of a brief talk on some aspect of the science program, followed by discussion. A feature of these informal seminars was that the climbers participated enthusiastically. This interest in the science shown by climbers continued throughout the expedition, and was indicative of the coherence of the two groups.

In retrospect, many of us believe that the scientific objectives of the expedition contributed a lot to our unity and sense of purpose. Climbers are intensely competitive, and on the usual type of expedition the climbers who reach the summit get most of the glory. The fact that others did an essential job in putting in the camps tends to be overlooked when the expedition is over. This attitude necessarily puts a tremendous premium on being a summiter, and highlights personal ambitions.

By contrast, our expedition had clear scientific objectives, and climbers who were not successful in reaching the summit made obvious contributions to setting up the laboratories and participating in the experiments. Moreover, the fact that no previous expedition had attempted to obtain scientific measurements at these extreme altitudes gave everyone a strong sense of purpose over and above that found on a regular climbing expedition.

After the expedition had ended I was surprised at the high level of interest in the medical research aspects from climbers in the American Alpine Club and elsewhere. Perhaps some of this stems from a hope that we have discovered some secret that will help climbers to tolerate altitudes. But in the main there just seems to be a great deal of interest in how high altitude affects the body. Incidentally, the compliment was returned during the afternoon following the big night avalanche, when Mike Weis and Jeff Lowe gave a seminar on snow conditions and avalanche risk.

The weather cleared on September 11, and the following day the climbers resumed their work on the icefall. That night Steve, Kop, Glenn, and Davey slept at the provisional Camp 1 site for the first time. Camp 1 was finally established on September 13, and soon only the scientists remained at Base Camp. The six-day delay caused by the storm forced us to take a hard look at the logistics of getting all the science loads up to Camp 2. Several people suggested that it would be better to send the Weatherport up to 2, and keep the rigid laboratory hut at Base Camp rather than the reverse, which was the original plan. This change would mean a substantial saving in carries because the Weatherport was only six loads whereas the hut was over thirty. Since it took two days to get a load from Base Camp to Camp 2, we were talking about a saving of at least forty-eight man-days.

Initially I objected to this change, partly on emotional grounds since so much time and money had gone into the design and testing of the laboratory hut, and there is no doubt that it would have been ideal at Camp 2. But I was eventually persuaded that another storm might so delay setting up the Camp 2 laboratory that the science would be at risk, so I agreed to the change of plan. In the event, the Weatherport turned out to be an excellent laboratory at Camp 2 and the reversal was a good decision.

At about this time I developed an illness that put me out of action for a few days. My right elbow suddenly became swollen, and Dave Graber diagnosed an olecranon bursitis (a bursa is a small sac of fluid around a joint that normally helps it to move). The infection rapidly spread until the whole arm from the wrist to the shoulder was red and swollen. It was initially treated with an oral antibiotic but it did not respond, and eventually I had to go down to Pheriche for a couple of days.

At these great altitudes minor infections often grumble on unless you descend to a lower altitude. Presumably the body's defenses are compromised by the low pressure of oxygen in the tissues, and so the healing process is abnormally slow. Duane Blume also went down at about this time because of infected cuts on his hand, and sherpa Ang Tshering as well because of an infected ulcer on his foot caused by an old leech bite that doggedly refused to heal.

Dave Graber prescribed intravenous cephalosporin (a powerful antibiotic) for me, and I was rather taken aback, considering this somewhat heroic. Fortunately Jim agreed to go down with me to give the injections. There was a nice jungle medicine scene when Jim gave me the first intravenous injection by candlelight in our tent at Base Camp at 2:00 A.M. There was another more hilarious occasion at Lobuya when, after a capital lunch of boiled potatoes which included several rounds of rakshi (an alcoholic beverage made by distilling potatoes), both Jim and I became rather tiddly and a Korean climber who happened to be staying in the hut there probably thought that I was some drug addict as Jim did his thing.

The two sherpas, Ang Tshering and Sungdare (not the same Sungdare who summited later), who accompanied Jim and myself down to Pheriche were an odd pair. Ang Tshering was suave, handsome, and very much a ladies man. He agreed to take my backpack because of my infected arm, and when we got to Lobuya, I found that a pretty sherpani was carrying his load! By contrast, Sungdare had a craggy face and rough manner, and we affectionately called him "neanderthal."

Once through the icefall, the climbers made their way up the very high but relatively flat valley, the Western Cwm, so named by Mallory in 1921 after the high valleys in north Wales. Here the terrain was much easier, but the climbers remained roped together because the valley was criss-crossed by snow-covered crevasses. The slope was gentle enough for some members to use skis in the Cwm.

Camp 2 was established on September 15, and every day after that a small army of sherpas would leave Base Camp at dawn and make their way up to Camp 1 at the top of the icefall with their 20-kg. (44-lb.) loads. At least they were supposed to be 20 kg., but the size of the load was decided by Sonam who cavalierly estimated the weight by briefly lifting it off the ground. One assumes that a sherpa who had incurred the sirdar's displeasure for some reason might end up with a somewhat larger load the following day!

I arrived back at Base Camp on September 19 with my arm well on the way to recovery. The news was good. Bob Winslow had completed all his Base Camp blood studies, and his equipment was packed and ready to go up to Camp 2. Larry Lahiri was in full swing with his scientific program; he was studying the control of breathing, and making measurements on sahibs and sherpas, both at rest and during exercise on the stationary bicycle. The climbers up high were moving fast.

John Evans had kept all the sherpas down at Base Camp so that they could be available for the big carry through the icefall. This was because our expedition was unique in terms of the huge amount of equipment that had to go above Base Camp chiefly because of the scientific laboratory at Camp 2. John had therefore arranged for all the cooking and other chores that are normally done by sherpas to be done by the climbers themselves at Camps 1 and 2. This unselfish attitude greatly helped in getting the two tons of food and equipment up to Camp 2.

At this time the climbers were starting to move up the headwall above the Cwm to find a site for Camp 3. The route John chose from the Cwm to the South Col was a direct line near the righthand edge of the southwest face of Everest. This approach was slightly to the right of the southwest buttress route used with great success by the Polish expedition in 1980.

This route had two advantages over the traditional route on the Lhotse face. One was that it was new ground and therefore more interesting and challenging from the climbers' point of view (though they did not anticipate any big surprises). In addition, the direct route was better for our scientific objectives. We planned to take blood samples at Camp 5 just above the Col, and then have these transported down to the main laboratory at Camp 2 within a few hours so that analyses could be made on the fresh blood. The samples would be placed on ice in a vacuum (Dewar) flask to slow down decomposition. We hoped this procedure would be feasible using the proposed route because a rope could be fixed the whole way from the Cwm to Camp 5, and sherpas or climbers could get down quickly. It would not have been possible to get blood samples down so rapidly via the longer Lhotse face.

The climbers were forging ahead at this stage, and I was even worried that they might get to the South Col before the scientists were ready for them. However, this turned out to be a needless concern.

On September 22 Jim and Rick left for Camp 1 on their way to set up the main laboratory at Camp 2. Those of us who remained at Base Camp got the remainder of the science loads ready for the last 900-meter (3,000-foot) ascent of their long journey from La Jolla. The various pieces of delicate electronic equipment such as the oxygen and carbon dioxide analyzers had been sent from California in custom-made padded packing cases. They did their job well but were too heavy to be taken up to Camp 2. So we simply wrapped the equipment in plastic foam, and arranged for the sherpas to carry it directly to

Camp 2 without a stop at Camp 1. This was a very long haul for one day but the sherpas could do it once the route was well beaten down, and they got paid extra for the double carry.

The sherpas were moving up the icefall very fast now. Typically they left in the morning at first light (about 5 A.M.) and were often back at Base Camp from Camp 1 by shortly after 9:00 A.M. having finished their day's work. The rest of us at Base Camp stayed in our sleeping bags until the morning sun hit the tents at about 8 A.M. Looking out through the tent door from the warmth of my sleeping bag I could see the sherpas as dots high in the icefall.

When they got back to camp the sherpas spent the rest of the day lounging about or betting on card games. These games could be quite noisy; the cards were thrown down with a defiant gesture and often a shout, but although the sherpas could argue fiercely, they almost never resorted to physical force in an argument.

On September 23 the advance climbers found a site for Camp 3 high on the headwall about 730 meters (2,400 feet) above the Cwm. The terrain was too steep to pitch the tents, but John had foreseen this problem, and Jeff Lowe had brought aluminum tubing and fabric to create platforms on which the tents could be placed. On one of the daily radio schedules I was asked to try to find this equipment in the Base Camp store, but I had no luck. However on the 25th, Brownie and Steve showed up at Base Camp. Steve was complaining of watery secretions in his lungs which kept him sitting up at night, and he thought that he had some kind of bronchitis. However this was almost certainly a form of high altitude pulmonary edema. I was embarrassed when Brownie immediately spotted the missing tent platforms in the store. We packed them so that they were ready to go up the following day, but they did not reach the Camp 3 site for over a week because of a delay that the expedition could ill afford.

September 26 was a big day for me; it was my turn to go through the icefall. The previous evening I wrote a quick note to my wife, Penny, just in case my night fears of the last few years came true. I was up at 4:00 A.M., and by the time we had had breakfast it was 5:15. As we left camp the sky was just lightening in the east, and a short time later the sun touched the top of Pumori giving it a bright tip. The dawn color was yellower than we see at sea level because the thin atmosphere at these altitudes does not scatter the blue wavelengths so much.

Peter Hackett was to shepherd Bob Winslow and myself through the icefall. I was surprised to find that all the wands that marked the route in the lower part of the trail had been knocked flat by wind blast from avalanches off the Lho La. It was tough going for me; although a rope had been fixed all the way to the top, some sections were very steep, and I was puffing like a steam engine. In some places crevasses 3 meters (10 feet) wide had been bridged by ladders, and these were tricky to cross, especially while carrying a pack. At times the route went perilously close (at least so it seemed to me) to the west shoulder of Everest on the left, and occasionally we crossed avalanche debris that straddled the trail.

After about two and a half hours we reached an area dominated by enormous seracs (ice towers). We came over a small hill, and stopped in utter astonishment. I remember Peter breaking out into a cackling laugh as we looked at the chaos in front of us. The route had been completely destroyed by an enormous collapse of ice. An area the size of several tennis courts had dropped down perhaps 20 meters (60 feet) leaving ladders at crazy angles, and ropes all awry. I looked at the desolation for a while stunned by the power of the icefall. We considered whether to try to climb around the disaster area, and took a few tentative exploratory steps, but the area still looked extremely unstable and hazardous. The sherpas adamantly refused to go on, and Peter decided that the safest thing to do was to return to Base Camp.

The implosion or collapse must have occurred during the previous afternoon or night because sherpas had used the icefall the morning before. Anyone who had been in the area at the time of the collapse would certainly have been killed. This is the closest I came to disaster during the whole expedition. I have thought about these events many times since, and there is really no way I can justify the risks of going through this icefall. As Peter said afterward, echoing Hillary, we wouldn't do it for any other mountain.

Bob and I went down together leaving Peter to explore ways of reestablishing the route. I was careful to retrieve my diary from my duffle bag; the bag was left by the route to be picked up on our next try. The trip down was tiring— the sun was blazing down, and with the absence of wind the icefall was like an oven. We did not arrive at Base Camp until 10:00 A.M., by which time I was utterly exhausted.

Snow fell that night and it was impossible to go into the icefall the following morning. However, I was glad to learn from the morning radio contact that Jim and Rick were going great guns setting up the Camp 2 laboratory. In addition, Larry had almost finished his exercise measurements, which meant that we could soon pack the bicycle and five of the solar panels in preparation for experiments to begin up at Camp 2. One serious problem was that the tent platforms that were destined for Camp 3 had been left in the icefall when we were unable to get through. In spite of this the climbers were pushing ahead, fixing ropes above Camp 3.

On September 29 there was a terrific storm. During the previous night I had heard an ominous continuous low-pitched distant roar caused by the wind up high, although there was very little air movement at Base Camp. In the middle of the night there was a tremendous avalanche that kept coming and coming, though it never reached Base Camp. We subsequently found that it had crossed the lower part of the icefall route, and it must have originated from very high above the Lho La on the west shoulder of Everest. It snowed all day at Base Camp, and the people at Camp 2 had a hard time of it. This storm swept the whole of the Himalayan range, and it was responsible for a number of expeditions being abandoned. Several climbers in other expeditions lost their lives as a result; we were lucky that none of our team was stranded above Camp 2.

Initially Kop and Davey had been at Camp 3, but they were able to get down before the storm became too severe. They and everybody else at Camp 2 sat tight in their sleeping bags to ride it out. The nylon roof was blown off the ice cave that served as a mess tent, and even the special tent that we had prepared for the scientific experiments at Camp 5 was damaged.

This last was a serious and unexpected blow. An enormous amount of time had been spent on the design of this tent to enable it to withstand the winds at Camp 5. These fierce winds, apparently the lower part of the jet stream, are funneled between the giant peaks of Everest and Lhotse, and the South Col receives the full fury. To our chagrin the tent had been damaged while erected in the much less exposed site of Camp 2.

October 1, certainly the most eventful day in my life for the last 20 years. We woke early; Big D, my tentmate, started packing his gear at 3:00 A.M. We were away at 4:45 before it was light using headlamps, and there was an eerie beauty about the icefall in the half-light. I got into difficulties almost immediately. We were crossing a frozen pool when the ice gave way, and I fell in with both feet up to the waist. Everything was soaking wet in an instant, but there was nothing for it but to go on. It took us about an hour to reach the bottom of the fixed rope, and then the magnitude of the day's problem became apparent. The rope was under several feet of snow, and had to be dug out almost all the way. In addition, the steps in the new snow were often as much as 2 feet deep, which made the going much more difficult. I soon bitterly regretted coming on this day when the trail had to be broken, and by 9:00 A.M. I was extremely tired.

My diary takes up the story. "Another disaster when we got up to the big serac area where we gave up last time. [Incidentally, I doubt if I had the energy for the trip back.] The arrangement was that eight sherpas would come down from Camp 1 to pick up the loads that had been left there—no sign of them. Very important because we had hoped that they would break the trail from there to Camp 1. I really wondered if I was going to survive the day. Extreme fatigue. Also, I knew we were in considerable danger from avalanches off the west shoulder—now 11 A.M. and the sun was beating down with a warmish wind. I constantly thought of Penny, Joanna, and Robert—this buoyed me up but frankly I was afraid I would die. Fortunately some sherpas did arrive from Camp 1 late in the piece—not only did they break trail but they took our packs. Nevertheless when I arrived at Camp 1 at 12:15 P.M. I was utterly exhausted.

"Met Davey Jones and Kop there—both in great form. Immediately sat down in the kitchen tent and had mugs of juice although strangely I had little thirst in spite of being obviously extremely dehydrated. Am sharing a tent with Bob—nice change. Surprised when I tried to take my boots off—they were stuck to my socks by the ice. The toes of both feet were quite white and numb. Peter Hackett was very concerned—he felt there was almost certainly a cold injury. He was for giving me morphine and putting my feet in a bowl of hot water (106 degrees F). However they improved in my bag and the warm water was not a bit painful. By the evening they looked fine although there was slight numbness at the ends of both big toes. [This numbness persisted for many months after the expedition.]

"Camp 1 is a magnificent site—glorious views over Pumori, Lindgren, Nuptse, Lhotse (the last does not look particularly high). I shall try some photography tomorrow.

"It seems that the reason why the Camp 1 sherpas did not appear is that a bridge across a crevasse was damaged and they turned back. There was in fact an easy route around this (which we had to take) though admittedly it went uncomfortably close to the west shoulder of Everest. Initially we had five sherpas with us but they also had to leave their loads in the icefall because they would not have been able to return to Base Camp in time if they had come right up to Camp 1. So now there are 13 loads in the icefall including the critical tent platforms. Another day lost to the high climbers—we may well pay dearly for this."

The next day was spent at Camp 1, and I was relieved to find that the additional altitude did not seem to be affecting me much. Chris Pizzo arrived having skied down from Camp 2; the terrain in the Cwm is sufficiently flat that it was possible to ski all the way from Camp 2 to Camp 1. After lunch Chris went down through the icefall alone, which seemed to me an unnecessary risk.

Saturday, October 3. Again, from my diary. "Another enormously exciting day—on to Camp 2. Somewhat restless night—first woke at 8:30 P.M.! Slept with inner boots in the sleeping bag to dry them . . . anyway bed tea at 5:30 A.M., then packed backpack and duffle (this ensures the absolute minimum for me to carry in the backpack!). Set off about 7:15—many delays with rope, ascenders, etc. There were four of us—Big D, Bob Winslow, Peter Hackett and myself. Great walk up to Camp 2. Sufficiently demanding that I was relieved when we arrived at 9:45 A.M. but what glorious scenery. First the top of Everest and the South Col hove into view (although the sun was directly ahead). Then many beautiful shots down the Cwm. What a privilege to be here. Terrific views of climbers going up the headwall to Camp 3—no question that the climbing difficulties increase an order of magnitude once you cross the bergshrund.

"Meeting with John and Duane. John expects summit bids in the window of October 12–18 (9–15 days away). This is a critical time . . . Lab now all ready to go for exercise runs. It will all happen in the next three weeks."

6

THE HIGHEST LABORATORY IN THE WORLD

"The griefe wee feele comes from the qualitie of the aire which wee breathe"[1]

Dawn on October 12 at Camp 2, 6,300 meters (20,700 feet) high. As I snuggle down as deeply as I can into my double sleeping bag I can hear some sherpas and climbers preparing to leave for their daily carry to Camp 3. I readjust the drawstrings of my Marmot bag so that my head is completely covered and there is only a thin tunnel of air leading to my nose. I am gradually getting the hang of all the controls on this thing. It is bitterly cold in the tent. The inside is covered with a rime of frozen water vapor, and an inadvertant bump sends it showering down on someone's face. The pee bottle that I used during the night is frozen hard. No sense in getting up just yet—I'll wait until the sun hits the tent, and the temperature starts to rise.

As I lie there I review the status of the expedition for the millionth time. The Camp 2 laboratory is going full steam ahead. We have many of the exercise experiments completed, and the sleep studies are coming along well. Duane and Bob have most of the blood samples that they need for their metabolism and hematology studies. Nine hundred meters (3,000 feet) below at Base Camp, Larry Lahiri has almost completed his experiments on the control of breathing. Nearly 1,800 meters (6,000 feet) above, the climbers are putting in Camp 5, the highest camp we shall have, and the takeoff point for the summit bids.

71

Everyone who is going to 5 has been thoroughly trained in the use of the equipment. Now all we need is lots of luck.

As I wriggle even lower into my womblike bag, I get a strong sense of security. However, I know that this is only partly justified. Although this site is relatively safe, it can be swept by avalanches from either the southwest face of Everest to the north or Nuptse to the south. I remember Chris Bonington's account of an avalanche that virtually flattened their camp in the same site in 1975. It had come down off Nuptse with a wind blast of devastating force, and although no one was killed, it reminded me that man is completely at the mercy of the elements here. A few days before we had seen an avalanche from Everest cross the trail between camps 1 and 2, but fortunately nobody was on the route at the time.

At last it is time for me to get up, pull on a few outer clothes, and shuffle over to the laboratory where Rick and Karl are already setting up for the day's work. The temperature in the Weatherport was -10° C. at 7 A.M., but it started to rise after the heater was coaxed into working. We had a great deal of trouble with the propane heater at Camp 2. It was not designed to work at such low oxygen pressures, and the main problem was getting it started. We sent off a long telex to the company in the U.S. via the ham radio linked to Kathmandu, but understandably they had never met this problem before and were not able to help very much. Eventually we determined that the heater could be started by blowing oxygen into it before it was lit. Then once it had warmed up it kept going under its own steam.

While the lab was warming up we all retired to the mess area for breakfast. This was a large ice hole dug out of the glacier and roofed with a nylon sheet. At the far end Kancha, our sherpa cook, did the best he could with a couple of propane stoves, and we sat on cardboard-covered ice benches. Breakfast and lunch were not so bad, but in the evening it could be bitterly cold, especially toward the end of October. The sun disappeared behind the great tower of Nuptse before 3 P.M., and that was a sign for the temperature in the valley to plummet. In fact, in the later stages of our stay at Camp 2 we all piled into the laboratory for the evening meal because the ice cave was so miserably cold.

With breakfast over it was time to visit the latrine, which was an open trench on the glacier 50 meters or so from camp. We always hoped that the call to this would occur while the sun was up; otherwise it was a frigid experience. Few people ventured off the two or three well-marked paths around Camp 2; you could never be sure where there was a hidden crevasse. We did not want a recurrence of the tragedy during the British Army Expedition of

1976. One of the climbers had got up during the night to relieve himself only to fall down a crevasse at Camp 2 to his death.

At 9 or so in the morning we started the day's experiments. The laboratory was busy from then until about 5 in the afternoon when we took a bit of a breather before the evening meal. Then there might be a card game in the lab while others read books. I found that my appetite for good books fell as the altitude rose, and at Camp 2 all I could handle were whodunits. It was humbling to recall that Mallory and Somervell read Shakespeare to each other when they shared a tent at the same altitude on the north side of Everest in 1922. By 8 P.M. or so most of us would retire for the night, and it was time to start setting up for the night's sleep experiment. This usually continued until about midnight.

One daily ritual was starting the gasoline generators to provide electrical power.[2] The chainsaw motors were very noisy, and they gave us a good deal of mechanical trouble. Various bolts sheared off during the course of the long, hard hours of work that they were given, and although we had spare motors, we were down to the last one by the time the scientific program ended. Rick and Karl did a terrific job keeping them going, though I sometimes wondered whether we might have saved ourselves some trouble by bringing in commercial generators. The main advantages of the chainsaw motors were that they are very light, and they have an enormous power output for their weight. They also have variable jets in the carburetors, and so can be adjusted for each altitude. They certainly gave their money's worth to our expedition.

The solar panels gave much less trouble being nonmechanical, and we were pleased with their performance. We had five of them up at Camp 2, and they put out a good 20 amps at some 15 volts under the intense radiation that poured into the Western Cwm. However, this was not nearly enough for our power-hungry laboratory particularly since the sun disappeared behind Nuptse in the early afternoon bringing the output of the panels to a sudden halt.

The rest of this chapter is devoted to a fairly nontechnical description of the research program at Camp 2. Any reader who would rather hear how the mountain was climbed should skip to the next chapter.

Figure 2 shows the chief research projects of the expedition.[3] Measurements were done at four sites, which were determined by the topography of Everest as approached from the south (compare the sketch of the mountain in Figure 1). The most extensive program was carried out in the main laboratory at Camp 2. In addition, however, several projects were completed in the Base Camp laboratory under the direction of Larry Lahiri. A few measurements were made at Camp 5, over 8,000 meters high. Finally, most ambitious of all, some

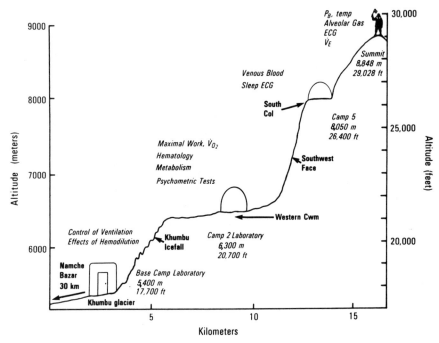

Figure 2.   The four sites on the mountain where medical research measurements were carried out. (Compare Figure 1, page 57.)

studies were planned for the summit itself (they are described in Chapter 8).

Much of our energy at Camp 2 was devoted to measuring the body's responses to exercise. As indicated earlier the primary physiological problem at high altitude is the reduced barometric pressure which means that the pressure of oxygen in the air is lowered. At Camp 2 the average barometric pressure was about 350 millimeters of mercury, as compared to the normal value of 760 at sea level. Therefore the oxygen was less than half the sea-level value. Actually, things are even worse than that. When air is inspired into the lungs, it is warmed and saturated with water vapor in the large airways. This water vapor displaces some of the inspired air with the result that the pressure of oxygen in the air as it enters the depths of the lungs is only about 63 as opposed to the normal sea-level value of about 150. As José deAcosta said back around 1600, "the griefe wee feele comes from the qualitie of the aire which wee breathe."

Oxygen is required by the exercising muscles for energy. When the body exercises, the oxygen consumption is greatly increased. At sea level a resting person consumes about 300 ml. (just over half a pint) of oxygen per minute, and the same is true at high altitudes. However, during severe exercise at sea level, the oxygen uptake increases up to about 15 fold. This enormous increase in oxygen demand in the face of the very low oxygen pressure in the air at high altitudes puts enormous stress on the oxygen transport system of the body. This includes the lungs, heart, and blood. How the body responds to these increased demands is one of the most interesting issues of physiology at extreme altitudes.

This topic particularly interested me. During the Himalayan Scientific and Mountaineering Expedition of 1960–61 we had carried out the highest exercise measurements to date. Not only did we complete an extensive program in the Silver Hut during the winter at an altitude of 5,800 meters (19,000 feet), but the stationary bicycle was taken to an altitude of 7,400 meters (24,400 feet) on Mt. Makalu, and we actually got measurements of maximal work capacity up there. They showed that the maximal oxygen uptake of the body at that altitude was only about 36 percent of its value at sea level.

Following the 1960–61 expedition we put together the available data on maximal oxygen uptake at various altitudes, and a very interesting result emerged.[4] Figure 3 shows that if we plot maximal oxygen consumption against barometric pressure (as the altitude increases, barometric pressure decreases) oxygen consumption falls off so rapidly at extreme altitudes that apparently almost no oxygen is available for useful work on the summit of Mt. Everest. The body needs oxygen to stay alive even when it is completely at rest; this is required to keep the vital organs such as the heart and brain functioning. Thus when Reinhold Messner and Peter Habeler reached the summit of Mt. Everest without supplementary oxygen in 1978, many physiologists including myself were astonished. Available measurements at somewhat lower altitudes strongly suggested that there was just not enough oxygen in the air.

This was one reason why we were so anxious to get good measurements of maximal work at Camp 2. Of course this was still a long way below the summit, but we had devised a way of obtaining information about exercise capacity on the summit in the relative comfort and safety of the Camp 2 laboratory. We did this by having the subjects exercise while they breathed from large bags (actually meteorological balloons) containing air with an abnormally low oxygen concentration. In other words, not only was the total pressure of the air reduced as a result of the high altitude, but we actually removed some of the normal amount of oxygen in the rarified air. This was done by the simple expedient of having subjects breathe air while pedaling at a comfortable rate on the stationary bicycle, and collecting what was exhaled. Since the exhaled air contained some carbon dioxide, which would have interfered with the experiments, this was removed by passing the air through soda lime absorbers. In

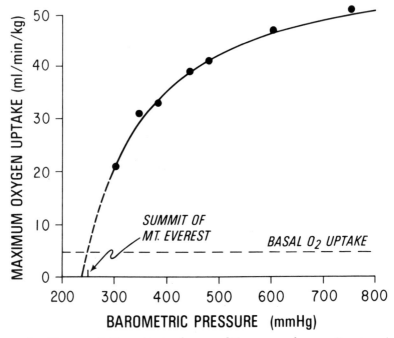

Figure 3. Data available prior to the expedition on work capacity at various altitudes. The maximal oxygen uptake, that is, the maximum amount of work that a climber can do, is plotted against barometric pressure. This pressure decreases as altitude increases. The points were obtained from measurements on acclimatized subjects. Note that extrapolation (extension) of the line indicates that almost all the oxygen uptake on the summit of Mt. Everest will be required for basal oxygen uptake, that is, the oxygen needed by the body without any physical activity. This suggests that a climber on the summit of Mt. Everest would be able to do almost no physical activity at all.

this way we prepared bags containing both 16 and 14 percent oxygen rather than the 21 percent that is in the air we normally breathe. Naturally anyone who had been eating garlic for breakfast was banned from this experiment!

The exercise testing consisted of the subject pedaling a stationary bicycle. It had a brake band on the wheel, and the tension could be adjusted and measured. It was a simple matter to calculate the amount of work that the subject was doing. For a particular exercise study he warmed up at a low work rate for several minutes, and then the load was increased to the desired level. He exercised at the given load for at least 3 minutes. During the last 2 minutes he breathed through a mouthpiece connected to a valve box so that we could collect all the exhaled air in a bag. The oxygen and carbon dioxide concentrations in the bag were measured using special electronic equipment, and we also measured the volume of the bag by expelling the air through a gas meter (a smaller version of the meter that measures the natural gas used by a house). The calculations needed to derive the oxygen consumption were on a programmable calculator to avoid arithmetical errors.

Some of our results[5] are shown in Figure 4. This time the oxygen consumption is plotted against the inspired oxygen pressure (PO_2) because this is what we changed. Notice that our members had appreciably higher maximal oxygen consumptions at sea level than those on the 1960–61 expedition. This goes along with the fact that our team had a number of marathon runners.

An important finding was that when the inspired oxygen pressure was very low our subjects showed a significantly higher oxygen consumption than the previous subjects. Although the difference was not great, it was sufficient to explain how Messner and Habeler could reach the summit. We found that the maximal oxygen uptake for the conditions on the summit was just over 1 liter per minute, a little less than a quarter of the sea-level value. However, by moving very slowly it should be possible to reach the summit with this oxygen uptake, severely limited though it is. With 1 liter per minute of oxygen uptake available, we calculate that a climber near the Everest summit would take 2 minutes to raise his own body weight (plus clothing and equipment) over a vertical distance of 10 meters. This is consistent with the climbing rates reported by Messner and Habeler. The reason why our measured oxygen uptakes were higher than predicted is explained by data we obtained subsequently on the summit, and is dealt with in Chapter 8.

While each subject was exercising, his heart function was monitored by recording his electrocardiogram. Resting heart rates are usually increased at high altitude, and on exercise the heart rate for a given level of work is higher. These changes may indicate that the heart's pumping action is reduced by the diminished oxygen supply since the amount of blood ejected for each heart beat is reduced. The heart rate during maximal exercise was lower compared with sea level, values of 140–150 per minute at Camp 2, whereas the value at sea level was 180–190. This change is partly accounted for by the lower maximal work rates at high altitude. We found very few abnormalities of heart rhythm.

Measurements of the amount of oxygen in the arterial blood were made by an ear oximeter. This works by shining a beam of light through the ear lobe, and measuring the color of the blood. As blood loses oxygen, its normal scarlet

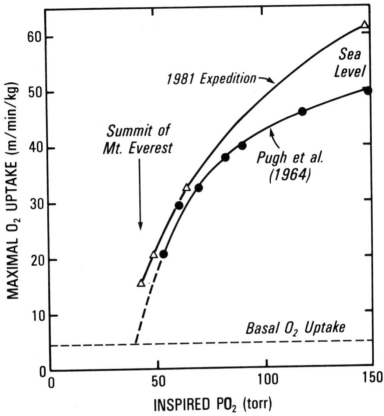

Figure 4. Maximal oxygen uptake plotted against the pressure of oxygen in the inspired air. The upper line shows the results obtained on this expedition. Note that although the maximal oxygen uptake (amount of work) that a subject can do when the pressure of oxygen is equivalent to that on the summit of Mt. Everest is extremely low, it is well above the basal oxygen requirements necessary to keep the body alive. This explains how Messner and Habeler were able to reach the summit without supplementary oxygen in 1978. The lower line shows the results available prior to this expedition. It is the same line as that in Figure 3 except that here the oxygen uptake is plotted against inspired oxygen pressure rather than barometric pressure.

color turns to blue, and thus it is possible to follow changes in the oxygen concentration of the blood. Invariably we found that the oxygen in the blood at rest was much lower than at sea level, and it became even lower during exercise. This indicated a failure of the normal transfer of oxygen in the lungs.

It turns out that under these conditions of extreme oxygen deprivation the lungs just do not have time properly to oxygenate the blood as it flows through them, and, as we say in technical jargon, oxygen transfer is "diffusion-limited."

A particularly striking example of this fall of blood oxygen was seen in Brownie Schoene when he performed maximal exercise while breathing 14 percent oxygen. The oximeter reading fell to the astonishingly low level of less than 10 percent, whereas the normal sea-level value is nearly 100. We began to wonder whether the extreme oxygen deprivation made this experiment too dangerous. But then we rationalized that since all the climbers and climbing scientists hoped to get to the summit where the pressure of oxygen in the inspired air was the same as it was in this experiment, they might as well be exposed to the hazard in the much safer environment of the Camp 2 laboratory! Incidentally, our whole experimental protocol had been given the green light by a special committee at the UCSD Medical School. This is a strict requirement of funding by the National Institutes of Health.

A number of sleep studies was carried out at Camp 2 and Base Camp. Some physicians and physiologists believe that whether or not an individual can tolerate these great altitudes may depend on the way he breathes during sleep. The nervous impulses from the brain that drive the breathing muscles tend to be fewer during sleep, and therefore the oxygen in the blood falls. In fact, the lowest levels of oxygen in the body at rest probably occur at night during sleep.

A striking feature of breathing during sleep at these altitudes is that it is very uneven.[6] This phenomenon is known as "periodic breathing" or "Cheyne-Stokes" breathing, and was first studied by the Italian physiologist, Angelo Mosso, at the beginning of this century. Mosso built the first high-altitude laboratory on the Monte Rosa in the Italian Alps, and there he noted that this type of breathing was very common—he even described it in his pet dog! Typically the subject breathes very deeply for a few breaths, and this is followed by several very shallow breaths or even no breathing at all. Initially it is a bit alarming to be sleeping in the same tent with someone who has marked periodic breathing; during the long breathing pause, you wonder if he is ever going to start again.

One of the most interesting features of this uneven breathing is that although almost all the westerners showed it, the sherpas generally did not. Larry Lahiri investigated this at the Base Camp laboratory, and he believes that it is probably related to the fact that, paradoxically, sherpas tend to breathe less than low-landers when the oxygen in the air is reduced. I say paradoxically because one might think that someone who is born and bred at a high altitude would have developed a larger breathing response to the low oxygen. But this is not the case. Larry believes that the lowlanders' large breathing response to low oxygen might cause instability in the control system during sleep. This phenomenon is well known to engineers who work with control systems.

For our sleep experiments the subject lay down in a special bunk in the laboratory while an observer kept an eye on him in the semidarkness. Various measurements were continuously recorded on a Medilog tape recorder, and from time to time a strip chart recording would also be made to check that the equipment was working properly. Breathing was measured with a thin wire vest worn next to the skin. Movements of the chest caused changes in the inductance of the vest, and could be written out on a pen recorder. At the same time we measured the oxygen in the blood using the ear oximeter. The oxygen level increased and decreased strikingly as a result of the changes in breathing; following each period of shallow breathing the oxygen would sometimes fall to less than half of its sea-level value. Other measurements included an electrocardiogram to see if the fluctuating oxygen levels affected the heart, and eye movements to determine how deeply the subject was sleeping. Occasionally we found that there were heart-beat irregularities when the oxygen fell to very low levels.

The only sherpa who showed periodic breathing was one of our liaison officers, Mingma. He lived in the village of Terhathum at an altitude of 1,500 meters (5,000 feet), considerably lower than Namche and the surrounding villages where most of our sherpas resided. Also, Mingma had spent several years in India at medical school, and it is possible that he had partially lost the adaptation to high altitude as a result of his long periods at lower levels.

Although the periodic breathing in the westerners was clearly related to the low oxygen of high altitude, the precise mechanism is not yet understood. However, Lahiri was able to show that when oxygen was administered during sleep, the breathing became more uniform, although some unevenness often still persisted. It was something of an experimental tour de force to change the inspired air while the subjects were sleeping, without waking them in the process; this was done using a specially constructed helmet. We were amused to learn from the firm that made the helmet that they had recently made a similar one for Clint Eastwood for the film *Firefox*.

Bob Winslow carried out an extensive series of blood studies;[7] he was assisted in this by Mickey Samaja who operated some of the very delicate equipment at Base Camp. We were reluctant to take this through the icefall, and instead brought the blood samples down to the equipment.

Some of the most obvious changes of the process of acclimatization to high altitude occur in the blood. For example, there is a large rise in the number of red blood cells, which are responsible for carrying the oxygen. This rise is brought about by stimulation of the bone marrow, which manufactures red blood cells, and means that the capacity of the blood to carry oxygen is increased. Our red blood cells increased by about 30 percent on the average, indicating a substantial response to the low oxygen. This was a smaller increase than on some previous expeditions, and we are not sure why. Perhaps our subjects were somewhat better hydrated; everyone was certainly kept aware of the importance of keeping up his fluid intake. Dehydration is a common problem at high altitude, and this would tend to raise the concentration of red cells.

We carried out an interesting experiment on the physiological benefits of these blood changes. It is usually assumed that the increase in red blood cells works to the advantage of the body because the increase raises the oxygen carrying capacity of the blood. Recently some physicians, however, especially in Europe, have argued that this change may be deleterious. The increased number of cells makes the blood thicker and more difficult to move, making the heart work harder, and probably causing some unevenness of flow in the very small blood vessels, which might interfere with the unloading of oxygen. These physicians advocate removing some of the blood, and replacing it with cell-free fluid. They argue that this "hemodilution" improves performance at high altitude, and lessens the risk of frostbite. However, a properly controlled study has never been done.

We tested the hypothesis in some experiments in the Base Camp laboratory near the end of the expedition.[8] Frank Sarnquist, Peter Hackett, and Brownie Schoene took the four expedition members who had the largest increase in red cells, removed some of their blood, and replaced it with cell-free human albumin solution (albumin is an important component of blood). The subjects were studied before and after hemodilution doing maximal work on the stationary bicycle, and psychological measurements were also made to see if brain function was altered.

Essentially no changes were found as a result of diluting the blood. The only significant difference was that heart rate (at a given exercise level) was increased following hemodilution; it is well known that heart rate increases when red-cell concentration falls. But there was no improvement in work capacity or brain function. Returning the blood nearer to its sea-level condition did not confer any advantage or disadvantage on the subjects of this study.

The result is interesting. It suggests that it is probably not justifiable to remove blood from climbers at high altitude as has been advocated, although it could still be argued that our tests did not cover all aspects of human performance.

But a more significant conclusion from a general biological point of view

81

is that the increased red-cell concentration was not an adaptive, but an inappropriate response to the low oxygen in the body. Physiologists often assume that because a particular physiological response occurs in some hostile environment, it must be adaptive. However, in this case it may be that the evolutionary pressure that resulted in this particular control mechanism (increased red cells as a result of low tissue oxygen) developed over thousands of years at sea level where the low tissue oxygen was caused by blood loss, and where the increased red-cell response would be truly adaptive. However, at high altitude, where the low tissue oxygen has a different cause (low oxygen in the inspired air) the red-cell response is inappropriate.

Bob Winslow and Mickey Samaja studied the acidity of the blood. A climber's breathing at high altitude increases tremendously, and this has the effect of making the blood very alkaline. We were astonished at the degree to which this happened, and it is discussed in more detail in Chapter 8.

Duane Blume, Jim Milledge, and Steve Boyer studied the chemical changes that occur in the body, including problems of nutrition. The low oxygen of high altitude seems to depress the function of many organs. In fact, some physicians liken living at high altitude to having some sort of chronic, grumbling disease; nothing is really working as well as it should.

For one thing, most people show a relentless loss of weight and this apparently occurs in spite of an adequate food intake.[9] On the Himalayan Scientific and Mountaineering Expedition of 1960–61 calorie intake was measured at an altitude of 5,800 meters (19,000 feet), and shown to be adequate for our level of activity. Nevertheless, everybody lost weight at the rate of 0.5 to 1.4 kg. (1 to 3 lb.) per week. The loss is not only fat; it is obvious from the spindly appearance of the arms and legs of somebody coming back from a high-altitude expedition that muscle substance is also lost.

Duane measured the ability of the gut to absorb xylose, a substance often used to test intestinal function. Absorption was abnormally low, presumably as a result of the reduced oxygen. He also measured the fat content of the feces in several subjects. This was increased, providing further evidence that the body was unable to extract nutrients from the food. Incidentally these fecal samples had to be diluted and then brought back to California in plastic bags for the analyses. This was obviously one of the less popular projects of the science program. There was an opportunity for a nosy U.S. Customs officer to get an unpleasant surprise, but happily this did not occur.

We studied many other of the body's chemical processes, but they are too technical to be described here. Duane, Jim, and Steve found a number of changes in the way in which the body handles carbohydrate, fat, and protein at these altitudes. For example, thyroid hormones increase, indicating that some chemical processes were being accelerated. [10] Other hormone changes suggested that the body was reacting to increased stress. In two subjects who both lost 15 kg. (33 lb.) over the course of the expedition, growth hormone was greatly increased, suggesting that the body was trying hard to repair the damage caused by the low oxygen. We also found changes in the chemicals that control body water, which may partly explain why water retention sometimes occurs. [11] Climbers sometimes develop puffiness around the eyes or swelling of the ankles, and the same mechanism may well be involved in high-altitude pulmonary edema and high-altitude cerebral edema.

None of these complicated analyses was done at Camp 2; this would have required too sophisticated a laboratory. Instead, the blood samples were frozen and brought back to the United States for analysis. Of course getting the frozen samples back was a tour de force. They were packed in liquid nitrogen and rapidly taken down to Syangboche just above Namche Bazar where they were flown out from a small landing strip. Actually, a few of them were inadvertently left behind in the freezer at Camp 2, causing some red faces, but these samples too were eventually successfully flown to the United States. It is very much to the credit of Duane and his colleagues that all the frozen samples eventually arrived in good condition.

Another series of studies was done on brain function at high altitude. [12] There is plenty of evidence to suggest that brain function may be affected at great heights. The mountaineering literature is full of examples of irrational decisions, many of which have led to disaster, and there have been a number of accounts of visual or auditory hallucinations. One was F. S. Smythe's account of pulsating cloudlike objects in the sky during the 1933 Everest expedition. He also reported a strong feeling that he was accompanied by a second person; the feeling was so strong that he even divided food to give half to his nonexistent "companion."

We had a package of psychometric tests put together by Dr. Brenda Townes and Dr. Tom Hornbein of the University of Washington. Tom Hornbein is a household name in American climbing. He was one of the five climbers to reach the summit in the first American ascent of Everest in 1963. His traverse with Willi Unsoeld up the West Ridge and down the Southeast Ridge was one of the triumphs of modern mountaineering, and is brilliantly described in his book, *Everest: The West Ridge*. Tom is now professor and chairman of the Department of Anesthesiology at the University of Washington Medical School. We had hoped that he would join our expedition as a scientist, but we had to settle for him as one of the Scientific Advisory Committee. His long interest in the effects of severe oxygen deprivation on brain function comes about through his work with patients who are anesthetized for long periods during difficult surgical operations. Together with Dr. Brenda Townes, a professor of psychology, he has done extensive studies in the psychometric function of these patients.

Brenda and Tom's tests for our expedition members were based on the Halstead-Reitan Test Battery that has been successfully used to assess the effects of drugs, trauma, and aging on brain function. Baseline studies were done before the expedition in La Jolla at the Veterans Administration Hospital, and a smaller group of tests was carried out at several altitudes on the mountain. These were administered by Brownie Schoene, also from the University of Washington. Immediately after the expedition Brenda flew out to Kathmandu, and did a series of followup studies there. A further series of tests was carried out at an expedition reunion twelve months later.

We were not surprised to find some impairment of mental function at camps 2 and 5. There was a tendency for the reduction in function to recover somewhat after the first couple of days at any altitude, indicating some sort of adaptation to the low oxygen. One of the tests that showed impairment was a test of short-term memory.

However, even more interesting was the fact that measurements made in Kathmandu immediately after the expedition showed some deterioration of mental function compared with the baseline studies made prior to the expedition. The largest change was in a finger-tapping test, a measurement of small-muscle coordination. There was also a significant impairment of short-term memory. This is one of the first clear demonstrations that a period spent at great altitudes causes alterations that persist when the subject returns to near sea level. These measurements were repeated a year later and, although the memory test had returned to preexpedition levels, motor coordination was still clearly abnormal in thirteen of the sixteen subjects. The precise mechanism for the deterioration in motor coordination is not understood, but one possibility is severe prolonged oxygen deprivation of the cerebellum, a part of the brain that controls muscular movement.

It should be emphasized that all our summit climbers used supplementary oxygen, and most climbers (though not all) started using oxygen at Camp 3, about 7,500 meters (23,800 feet). The results might give pause to climbers who plan to go very high, especially without supplementary oxygen. The degree of oxygen deprivation is so severe under these conditions that residual effects on brain function are not at all surprising. Perhaps the only real surprise is that it has taken so long to document the deterioration.

The chief reason why we did not make a lot of measurements on the sherpas is that the expedition was designed to obtain data on lowlanders at extreme altitudes. As interesting and important as these data would be, a much less elaborate expedition would have been suitable for this, and indeed there have been research expeditions concentrating on sherpa physiology. Larry Lahiri and Jim Milledge have taken part in some of them.

However, we did make measurements on sherpas at Base Camp—the measurements of breathing during sleep have already been discussed—and Bob Winslow did some blood measurements on the sherpas near the end of the expedition.[13] Previous reports have suggested that sherpa blood is considerably different from that of both acclimatized lowlanders and permanent residents of high altitude in the Peruvian Andes. However, Bob found that this was not the case. There does not seem to be any marked difference between sherpa blood and that of the Andean natives. The previous anomalous results can probably be explained by the fact that blood samples were taken long distances before they were analyzed, and this introduced errors.

The last study is one of the most interesting. Larry Lahiri and Brownie Schoene made extensive measurements on the increase in breathing that occurred when the oxygen concentration in the inspired air was deliberately reduced.[14] Physiologists refer to this as the "hypoxic ventilatory response," "ventilation" meaning the amount of air that is moved by the lungs, that is, the volume of each breath multiplied by the number of breaths per minute. It has been known since the early part of the century that if the amount of oxygen in the air is reduced, the breathing increases. This increased ventilation is brought about by small sensors or "chemoreceptors" located on arteries going to the brain. These sensors detect the reduction in oxygen in the blood, and send nervous impulses to the brain with the result that more nervous impulses go to the muscles of respiration thus stimulating increased breathing.

There are considerable differences between individuals in the extent to which their breathing responds to low oxygen. This is genetically determined, like eye or hair color. Larry and Brownie were particularly interested in whether this breathing response to low oxygen correlated with performance at high altitude. There had been previous intimations that this might be the case.

Several interesting conclusions emerged from their studies at sea level, Base Camp, and Camp 2. First, it was clear that the ventilatory response to low oxygen at sea level was a good predictor of the increase in ventilation at high altitude. Moreover, this applied not only to ventilation at rest, but also during exercise. But the most interesting finding was that there appeared to be a strong correlation between an individual's ventilatory response to low oxygen, and his climbing performance or tolerance to high altitude. In fact, if we ranked the expedition members by their hypoxic ventilatory response as measured by Brownie in Seattle, it turned out that the climber with the highest response got to the summit first, the one with the next highest got to the summit second, and the one with the third highest got to the summit third (Figure 5). In addition, those individuals who were born with a low ventilatory response to low oxygen generally tolerated the extreme altitudes bjadly.

An example of the handicap of a low hypoxic ventilatory response was John Evans, who had one of the lowest values. As climbing leader he naturally wajnted to climb as high as possible. But on the two occasions when he went to Camp 3 (7,250 meters, 23,800 feet), he developed splitting headaches, nausea, and on one occasion uncontrollable retching. It was clearly impossible for him to sleep there, much to his disappointment. Of course this was no indictment of his moral fiber; the fact is that he was born with an unusually small ventilatory response to low oxygen, and at extreme altitudes this is as much a physical handicap as a broken leg.

The physiological advantage of a vigorous response to low oxygen at high altitude is clear. The increased breathing raises the level of oxygen in the air

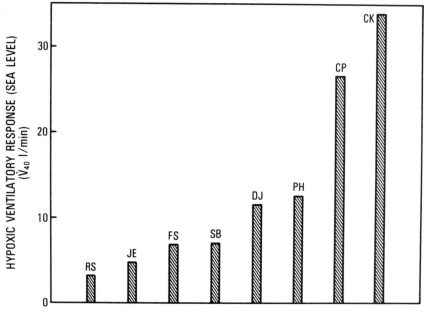

Figure 5.   The hypoxic ventilatory response, that is, the extent to which subjects increase their breathing when given a low-oxygen mixture to inhale at sea level, for various members of the expedition. It turned out that the subject with the highest response, CK, reached the summit first. The subject with the second highest response, CP, reached the summit second, while the third highest responder, PH, reached the summit third. In general there was a good correlation between the response and performance at extreme altitude.

in the depths of the lungs, and this tends to make up for the reduction of oxygen in the inspired air. Other things being equal, this means a higher level of oxygen in the arterial blood. Interestingly, this correlation does not hold in some other sports. Brownie has shown that the best middle-distance runners and competitive swimmers tend to have a low breathing response to low oxygen. In these instances the additional energy required to cause increased movements of the respiratory muscles may be a disadvantage. Certainly there is little point in raising the level of oxygen in the air in the lungs in these competitors because there is plenty of oxygen available at sea level.

The advantage of a large breathing response to low oxygen is really seen only at extreme altitudes, say, above 6,500 meters (21,000 feet). Thus the phenomenon is probably not important to the rock climber in the California Sierra or to the recreational trekker.

A corollary of this work is that for the first time we have a way of predicting performance at high altitude. This has been one of the bugbears of the selection of climbers for Himalayan expeditions in the past. Generally it is argued that the only reliable predictor is whether someone has been high before, and certainly that is still a good criterion. But it obviously cannot be universally used otherwise no one would be selected for the first time.

Our measurements suggest that at the very least it should be possible to identify individuals who may not do well at extreme altitudes, that is, people born with a low breathing response to hypoxia. This measurement is easy to make in any pulmonary function laboratory. Of course the endowment of a vigorous breathing response to low oxygen does not ensure good performance at extreme altitudes; other factors such as physique and fitness come into the equation. Also, as Hillary's foreword to this book reminds us, motivation is a sine qua non.

There is a paradox here: the sherpas tend to have a reduced breathing response to low oxygen, and yet they perform extremely well up to altitudes of 7,500 meters (24,500 feet) or so. It must be that our relatively crude measurements cannot determine everything that is going on at the tissue level. A sherpa who has adapted through many generations to the low oxygen of high altitude has developed subtle cellular changes that enable him to perform well despite a low level of oxygen in the lungs. A corollary of this is that "acclimatization," the process of change that occurs when lowlanders go to high altitudes, is not necessarily the same as the true adaptation to high altitude that is seen in permanent residents over the course of generations.

How can we summarize the results of all these studies at Camp 2 and Base Camp, and what does it all mean for the average climber who wants to improve his performance? Many of our findings are technical, and since they are at the cutting edge of medical research, some of the implications are still not clear.

However, our scientific program has documented the very broad deterioration in body function that occurs at great altitudes. The body's ability to do work was greatly impaired. At Camp 2 laboratory maximal work levels were about one-half those at sea level, and when we simulated conditions on the Everest summit, work levels were down to less than a quarter of the sea-level control. From the point of view of a useful engine, the body is slowly grinding to a halt as it goes higher.

This reduced work capacity is directly attributable to the very low levels of oxygen in the air and therefore in the exercising muscles. This oxygen deprivation is also reflected in the very low levels of oxygen in the blood, particularly during exercise. The lungs were just not built for these conditions or, more accurately, the centuries of evolutionary change at sea level have not produced lungs that can function properly at these extreme altitudes.

Sleep was another affected function. The normal control of breathing was disrupted by the low levels of oxygen, and breathing became uneven or periodic. As a consequence, the oxygen level in the arterial blood plummeted following the phases of reduced breathing, and it may well be that these very low levels of oxygen during sleep play a major role in determining who can tolerate great altitudes. Certainly many climbers who sleep without supplementary oxygen at altitudes of over 7,000 meters (23,000 feet) complain that they wake feeling drained rather than refreshed.

The sherpas generally do not have the same problem during sleep, and this appears to be one example of how being born and bred over generations at high altitudes has improved the body's adaptation to low oxygen.

We saw marked changes in the physiology of the blood. These included a striking increase in the number of red cells, the elements of the blood responsible for carrying oxygen, and also a marked alkalinity, which can be explained by the increased breathing in response to the low oxygen. However, the increased number of red cells was of questionable value. When the red-cell concentration was reduced to nearer the normal level by removing blood, there was no reduction in work capacity or brain function. This suggested that the increase in red cells was an inappropriate response to the low oxygen of high altitudes, whereas it clearly has a useful role at sea level if the oxygen deprivation of the body tissues is caused by anemia.

Another conclusion of our study on hemodilution was that there seems to be no justification for removing blood from climbers at high altitudes, as has been advocated by some physicians. We found no improvement in the function of the heart, lungs, or brain.

Extensive changes in body chemistry were demonstrated as a result of the oxygen deprivation. Many of these are technical, and the full implications of some are not yet clear. However, we believe that the body is responding to the increased stresses of high altitudes in various ways, but nevertheless oxygen deprivation results in deterioration in many areas. Absorption of food is reduced, partly accounting for weight loss. Hormonal controls are affected. The control of water balance is altered, and this may contribute to high-altitude pulmonary edema and cerebral edema.

The brain functions less efficiently at these altitudes. This in itself is not surprising; it is well known that the brain needs lots of oxygen for normal function. What was surprising was the clear demonstration of residual impairment of brain function following the expedition. Both short-term memory and motor coordination were affected, though the former returned to the preexpedition levels within twelve months. By contrast, motor-coordination abnormality was present in a majority of the expedition members one year after our return to sea level, and the clear implication is that a prolonged period of exposure to the very low levels of oxygen at great altitudes can cause deterioration of brain function for some time. Climbers who plan ascents of 8,000-meter peaks without oxygen should keep this in mind.

Finally, measurements on the extent to which people increase their breathing when the oxygen in the air is reduced suggest that we may have a useful predictor for who can tolerate these great altitudes. The "hypoxic ventilatory response" varies considerably among individuals, and is genetically determined. We are born with it, and there is nothing that we can do to change it. Our measurements clearly showed that climbers with a relatively low hypoxic ventilatory response tended to tolerate extreme altitudes poorly. This may be a useful guide to selection of climbers for expeditions to extreme altitudes.

Large areas of ignorance still remain about how the body functions at high altitudes. Although our research program was extensive, almost no studies were devoted to the changes that occur at the cellular level. We recognized the importance of this part of the body; after all, that is where the oxygen is actually utilized. The chief problem is that many studies of cell function can be made only by invasive measurements such as biopsies (taking samples of tissue with a needle, for example), and it is difficult to justify such procedures on a field expedition. Thus, although a lot has been learned from our research program, much more needs to be done.

7

SUMMIT!

"A single, narrow, gasping lung,
floating over the mist and summits"[1]

When John Evans accepted the position of climbing leader way back in 1977, relatively little thought had been given to the route. As planning developed, it became clear that our scientific objectives imposed a number of constraints, and we realized that the traditional South Col route, or some variant of it, had a number of obvious advantages.

One of our principal goals was to obtain physiological measurements at altitudes over 8,000 meters (26,200 feet), and one way of doing this was to have a small scientific camp near the South Col where climbing scientists could be based. They would then be able to make measurements at this camp and, just as important, help to attach instruments to the climbers who would go from this top camp to the summit. Well into the expedition we clung to the strategy of having a team of four sahibs at Camp 5 at any time; one pair would be the climbers poised for a summit bid with or without sherpa support, while the other pair would consist of climbing scientists who prepared the climbers to make the proper measurements, and collected the data when they got back to Camp 5.

Toward the end of September we realized that this tidy plan was coming unstuck. The weather conditions had become so ferocious on the Col that we were fast running out of climbers and climbing scientists who were fit enough to make a summit bid. Having two climbing scientists at Camp 5 who were not supposed to go any higher meant that the chances of anyone getting to the summit were substantially reduced. This made no sense.

Another important feature of the expedition design that affected the route was the siting of the main laboratory camp. Although we planned an extensive research program there, an equally important function of this laboratory was as a logistical support base for the physiology at extreme altitudes. We needed to make final tests on the physiological equipment that the summiters would take. We also needed to prepare the ampules for the alveolar gas measurements to be made at Camp 5 and above, and test the stationary bicycle that we originally hoped to use at Camp 5. Even more important, blood samples taken at Camp 5 were to be analyzed by Bob Winslow using equipment at the main laboratory camp.

These considerations dictated that the main laboratory be relatively high in the Western Cwm, and that there should be rapid access from Camp 5 down to the laboratory. As indicated earlier, a happy solution to all these problems was John's choice of a direct route from the Cwm to the South Col on the buttress forming the right-hand (south) edge of the southwest face. This was just to the left of the slope used by Miura, the man who skied down Everest. This route for the 1,700 meters (5,500 feet) between camps 2 and 5 had the additional advantage that the climbers were on new ground for part of the way, although they were not far to the right of the route used by the Poles in 1980.

Another requirement for Camp 2 was a relatively large flat area for the science laboratory and associated equipment. This was easily found in the upper part of the Western Cwm. This choice of site for Camp 2 meant in turn that the expedition was committed to the traditional icefall route and also the traditional site for Base Camp.

Early in the science planning we did not see the point of having a laboratory at Base Camp. However, it became clear that it would be too difficult to move some of the delicate equipment through the icefall, and that some important measurements (mainly on blood samples) could be done the day after they had been brought down through the icefall. Just as important, it would be essential to have spares of all the scientific equipment, and we reasoned that since the equipment would be there, why not use it for an additional research program at Base Camp.

This was an excellent decision. Most of the pieces of equipment in the Camp 2 laboratory were duplicated at Base Camp, and we could always move a piece of equipment up if something critical failed. If ever there is a situation where redundancy of equipment is justified, a scientific expedition to Everest is it. Additionally, one of our most profitable decisions was to invite Larry Lahiri to carry out a research program in the Base Camp laboratory. Larry is an eminent high-altitude physiologist, and his program contributed greatly to the scientific productivity of the expedition. Another fortunate feature of this arrangement was that he planned to do some measurements on sherpas, and this fitted well with his location at Base Camp. At Camp 2 we could devote ourselves entirely to measurements on the acclimatized lowlanders.

It turned out that our scientific objectives and the route that John chose fitted beautifully. The topography of the mountain as approached from the south lends itself extremely well to this type of medical scientific expedition, the only serious disadvantage being the danger associated with the icefall. I shall be very surprised if some other group does not take advantage of this experimental design again within the next few years.

In February 1980 John put together twenty pages of climbing plans. These included two extensive tables showing the progress of the climbers, scientists, and sherpas from Base Camp to Camp 2, and from Camp 2 to the summit. For each day the chart showed the number of people at each camp, the activity for that day, and the disposition of all the loads. A number of alterations were made to this preliminary plan in May 1980, and a final climbing plan was prepared in April 1981.

Some general principles emerged from these plans. The icefall was going to be a substantial bottleneck in terms of the number of loads that had to go through it in a limited time. John calculated that a total of 3,640 kg. (8,000 lb.) had to be lifted through the icefall within 10 days of the route being opened, and at 20 kg. a load this was over 180 man-days of carries. This of course was a direct result of having the sophisticated and heavy laboratory at Camp 2. Very early John decided that the best way to beat this problem was to prepare the icefall route as soon as possible, and to use only small teams of climbers to carry out a reconnaissance in the Cwm while everybody else was doing carries through the icefall. This plan worked well, though it was tough sledding for the climbers in the Cwm to make do without sherpa support for a couple of weeks.

It was not until September 23 that sherpas began to occupy Camp 2, even though it had been sited on the 13th. By the 23rd the climbers had carried 51 loads up to Camp 2, fixed lines to Camp 3 at an altitude of 7,250 meters (23,800 feet), and even made 7 carries to Camp 3 in anticipation of moving further up on the following day. By this time the sherpas had carried 250 loads through the icefall, and taken over the task of carrying between camps 1 and 2.

On September 24 John Evans and Davey Jones moved up to Camp 3. The chosen site had excellent avalanche protection under a large overhanging rock, but the snow and ice surface was too steep to pitch a tent. This problem had been anticipated, and the expedition had brought in aluminum platforms on which tents could be erected. These were partially in place by the 24th, but more were needed so a radio message was sent down to Base Camp where they were stored. At this time John was having trouble with the altitude, which caused a severe headache and some retching, so he descended to Camp 2 while Kop went up to join Davey at 3.

During the next two days Kop and Davey fixed ropes above Camp 3, reaching the site of Camp 4 at about 7,500 meters (24,500 feet). The sherpas were now making daily carries to Camp 3, and the climbers were optimistic that they would be on the South Col by the end of the month. This was excellent news. The weather was likely to deteriorate by mid-October as a result of high winds and very low temperatures. Being poised for the summit assaults at the beginning of October was ideal timing.

Our optimism turned out to be short-lived. As indicated earlier, a violent windstorm on September 27 raked the Western Cwm and above, and Kop and Davey were forced to move back down to Camp 2. Over the next couple of days Camp 2 rode out a terrific storm. It did not do a great deal of damage, but we were chagrined that the special tent prepared for the science laboratory at Camp 5 was torn. This Bishop Ultimate tent had been strongly reinforced in preparation for the anticipated high winds above the South Col, and it was a big blow to find that it was not able to withstand a storm in the relative shelter of the Western Cwm.

Incidentally, when I got back to Kathmandu and spoke to Elizabeth Hawley about the successes and failures of expeditions during the fall, she told me that a number were abandoned as a result of this storm, which swept the whole of the Himalayan range, and that several climbers died. Relatively little snow settled at Camp 2 because of the high wind, but the icefall and Base Camp were covered with about 60 centimeters (2 feet) of snow. This was the snow that gave me so much trouble getting through the icefall.

The tent platforms finally got to Camp 3 on October 3 in a big carry led by Frank and Jeff with a strong group of sherpas. The steep terrain there caused a problem because it was difficult to find enough space or hanging points to secure the loads and stop them tumbling down back into the Cwm. However, on October 5 Glenn and Jeff established Camp 4, and during the next two days they fixed ropes to very near the South Col. Just above Camp 4 they deviated from the Polish route that continued directly up to the south summit bypassing the Col. Instead Glenn and Jeff headed to the right toward the southeast ridge. They moved up a steep snow field to the left of the Geneva spur on a route that would meet the southeast ridge about 60 meters (200 feet) above the South Col at an altitude of 8,050 meters (26,400 feet). This would be the site of Camp 5.

Although the weather at Camp 2 remained mostly fair, fierce winds near the Col made establishing Camp 5 difficult. Steve Boyer and Dave Graber worked on the route above 4, and eventually a feasible site for Camp 5 was found by Steve, nestled under a sheltering rock cliff. By now it was October 10, and time was beginning to slip through our fingers.

That same day the first "summit team" of Davey Jones, Chris Kopczynski, and Chris Pizzo moved up to Camp 3 with three sherpas. Theirs was a very optimistic plan—complete fixing rope to Camp 5, establish and occupy that camp, and subsequently make a summit bid. They established the camp the following day, though the sherpas were feeling the effects of the altitude. The three climbers and two sherpas then stayed at Camp 5 for three days in the hope of making a summit attempt, but the high winds made this out of the question and eventually forced them to retreat to Camp 2 on October 14. Nevertheless, the time was not wasted. Chris took alveolar gas samples on Davey, Kop, and himself, and also made a measurement of barometic pressure. The value of 282.1 was about 2 mm. mercury higher than I had predicted, and this was the first indication that we had underestimated the pressure on the summit.

At this stage there was serious concern about whether we had left the summit bid too late. A second potential summit team consisting of Glenn Porzak, Frank Sarnquist, Peter Hackett, and Yogendra Thapa (one of our liaison officers now promoted to full climbing responsibilities) moved up to Camp 3 on the morning of the 14th. It was very disappointing for those of us at Camp 2 that the weather high on the mountain was very fine and still on the 15th, but of course there was no one at Camp 5 to take advantage of this and make a summit assault. Frank had a bad night at Camp 3, and decided to make a quick carry up to Camp 5 and then descend. Glenn, Peter, and Thapa sorted out loads at Camp 3, and then climbed to Camp 5. However, they arrived too late to make a summit bid on the 16th, though they reported that the weather was almost feasible.

The weather now deteriorated again, and this time the winds increased to hurricane force. During the night of the 16th all but one of the tents at Camp 5 was destroyed, and this second proposed summit team had to abandon Camp 5 and return to Camp 2. Glenn Porzak arrived back at 2 during lunchtime looking absolutely beaten. His voice was all but gone, but he managed to recount a desperate story of the descent from Camp 5.[2]

"The winds started to pick up around 11 o'clock last night, but notwithstanding we got up at about 1:30 A.M. and I went out and talked to the sherpas and they agreed that they would make a carry for us today. Even though the wind steadily increased we continued to get ready, I guess on some foolish hope that it would all of a sudden die down. Peter connected up my Medilog recorder, but he connected the wrong button so I had to open up my chest to him on two occasions at 3 o'clock in the morning at over 26,000 feet and it was an ordeal to say the least. But we managed to get ready with some tea brewed, and I ate my favorite pop tart which gave me great nourishment. [Glenn had some dietary idiosyncrasies.]

"At about 4:30 A.M. we got up, and I went outside and was greeted to the wind blast of my life. I couldn't believe the velocity. I had my complete oxygen gear on, and the wind was so strong that it somehow interfered with the use of the diluter demand system. I stood out there probably for about four or five minutes just kind of in awe of the situation. There was this enormous jet stream—it was flying directly overhead—and there was an incredible wind plume on Lhotse.

"I went over and talked to the sherpas, and we immediately agreed that there was no way there could be any summit attempt today, so we went back into our respective tents and decided that maybe we could wait things out for a while. If nothing else, we could perhaps make a carry of oxygen loads so as to take that problem away. We might have been able to carry them up perhaps to 27,500 feet.

"But as the morning progressed it just got steadily worse and worse. It must have been about 8 or 9 o'clock when we quickly realized that it had turned into kind of a critical situation, that it was just a matter of time until maybe the tents would start going, and that we ought to start thinking about some sort of evacuation.

"We tried on a couple of occasions to dig out our old Dunlop tent. Doing that made a great impression on me. It's not like digging out a tent down there at Camp 2. Just a little effort, and we would just sit there and be gasping for breath in the incredible winds. You could only be out there for so long, and then you had to come in gagging for breath.

"And then early morning turned into late morning and early afternoon, and the winds were of just unbelievable velocity, and it was all we could do to keep half of the tent propped up while the other guy was trying to get his stuff packed. We finally got out of there somewhere around noon, and I chose to go without oxygen. Peter said he was going to use oxygen. However, he later told me that he experienced the same thing with the wind when it affected the diluter demand system. He got out to start to go down, and he just ran back to the tent and stripped off all his oxygen gear!

"For me personally, the winds were coming straight up the fixed line, and my great compliments to Steve, Davey, and Jeff for fixing that upper 1,000 feet or so. You couldn't look into the wind. I came down absolutely with my eyes closed, and just kind of hand over hand looking at the line only to change the karabiner or jumar. That's the honest truth. There's no way you can protect your eyes in that kind of situation. That is really about it; it was hellacious coming down."

Glenn's voice remained husky for several days, and although he stayed at Camp 5 until the 20th he never fully recovered his strength. It was remarkable how a short period under these extreme conditions could so weaken a strong man. Thapa was so exhausted by the gale that he was unable to get down to Camp 2, and instead spent the night of the 17th at 3.

On the night of October 17 Jeff Lowe shared my tent. Jim Milledge had moved down to Base Camp the previous day because he had finished his measurements. Also, since he had been on Bonington's expedition to Kongur in China in the spring and had spent only one week with his family in between expeditions, he was understandably yearning for the comforts of home. Jeff was up at about 2 A.M. to have breakfast with Mike Weis, Kop, and Steve, and they all headed up to Camp 3. I learned later that Jeff and Mike hoped to make an oxygenless ascent; I think if I had known this I would have tried to dissuade them because at this stage it looked as though we would get no data at all above Camp 5.

The four climbers were held up at Camp 4 for a day by high winds. The following day took a toll; both Steve and Jeff became very short of breath, and in retrospect both of them probably had early high-altitude pulmonary edema. This was the second time that Steve developed evidence of this condition. The first was when he arrived back at Base Camp on September 25 complaining of watery secretions in his lungs; this was almost certainly a form of pulmonary edema. It was very bad luck for Steve; he drove himself hard, and was certainly one of the most highly motivated members of the expedition. Nevertheless, like everybody else who helped with the high carries but did not make the summit, he made an essential contribution to the ultimate success of the expedition.

When Mike, Kop, and the sherpas arrived at Camp 5 they found only a single tent standing, the others having been destroyed by the gale force winds above the Col. Mike decided to withdraw, feeling that Kop and Sherpa Sungdare looked very strong for a possible summit bid the following day.

October 21. A red-letter day for the expedition, although down at Camp 2 there was little information about what was going on. Radio contacts with camps 3, 4, and 5 had been virtually nonexistent for the last couple of days for reasons we did not fully understand. The chief problem was probably that the batteries lost their punch unless they were kept warm inside a sleeping bag. Fortunately we have a good firsthand account from Kop that he dictated into a tape recorder on the day that he returned to Camp 2, and I shall let him take up the story on the evening of the 20th.

"I went out and started digging around for the science gear, for the barometer—I couldn't find it. You know how it looks in a tent just packed with ice. So I got in and I started cooking, and about an hour later I said 'Sungdare, this respirator doesn't work'—it was a Blume one. And I had one Hornbein, and I said we need to find another one for you—I will cook, and you go out and look in between the tents and everything. The next thing I knew I heard this ripping noise. He'd taken his axe to that VE24 tent—it was full of snow anyway—and just started pulling the side and guts out of it and he found it way in the back. In about 45 minutes I was going to tell him to forget it, I'll take the Blume, and if it works, fine. If it doesn't . . . it was kind of . . . you couldn't tell if it was working or not. He found it and then we went . . . I got out and looked around inside that tent for the science gear. I couldn't find anything, and then I found out yesterday that Peter said they stuffed it all into the Dunlop tent!

"Well, anyway after that . . . that was about 7 at night. The winds were oh, about 40, just a constant 40 mile an hour wind. I just told him, tomorrow we've got to talk no matter what, you know, no matter what the winds. I had some extra clothing that the sherpas took up—an extra jacket. Sungdare complained that his feet were cold, and it was kind of cold, so I gave him my down jacket and an extra pair of pants. He was pretty happy about that—he put those on. And then his feet . . . you know, there's no toes. He's got one little bitty toe about that big, but he put a pair of socks on, and he put the boot on, and he put an extra pair of socks over the boot, and got it really . . . I had some extra socks up there too, luckily. [Sungdare had lost 9 toes through frostbite on the 1979 German Everest expedition.] So things were starting to fall into place a little more. My partner was up to this thing . . . because both people have to be or . . . forget it.

"Anyway, he got all warm, and he said 4 o'clock you wake me and I'll make tea. I said, no, 3 o'clock. He says, no, 4 o'clock. I said, okay Sungdare, 4 o'clock. We'll leave at 6.

"Well, it's impossible to start at 4, and leave at 6. All night long we both slept in an L-shape because the tent was so pushed around with snow that you just sit like this and try to sleep. Sungdare could sleep, I couldn't. Then at 3 I tried to trick him into thinking it was 4, and woke him up. He wanted to look at my watch . . . it was really 3. We did come to a compromise. At a quarter to 4 we started cooking. The wind was still just a constant 45 miles an hour I'd say, average, and it just looked like we were going to go through some motions, go out and get cold, and come back. I said that the least we could do was carry an oxygen bottle each up to 27,500, and then the next party will have the oxygen up there. Well, then, as the reality came, it came to 6 o'clock and we weren't ready. I started to put on my crampons, and I got outside. I had to splice a piece of rope . . . it was so tangled up . . . I couldn't find a knife so we cut it with an axe. I was so cold and so winded after that hour of working outside in the morning. I was already getting thirsty again, and since we had only one water bottle between us we decided just go for it.

"I just put one bottle of oxygen in my pack, and hooked up and started up the slope. Sungdare waved to me and said, 'Do you want me to carry the oxygen, an extra bottle?' I said, if you can. Carry it as far as you can. So he stuck an extra bottle in, and we started up the slope at exactly 7 o'clock.

"We went about 20 minutes in just incredible winds at the South Col. The winds just started cutting you into the core. The sun was out though, and we could see well and everything. We went around the corner about another 20 minutes up into those gullies, and all of a sudden it just started getting gusty— you know, you'd have a calm, and then you'd have a gust. I felt a tug on the rope, and turned around, and Sungdare was taking the bottle of oxygen out of his pack. He just stuck it into the snow. So I looked at that, and just kept going.

"We got about 500 feet above the Col, and you could have taken out your thick liner. Then Sungdare stopped. He had kind of a smile on his face, and he pulled out his gloves like this, and both of them fell out of his hand, and they went down the slope. So I thought, well, this is the start of a good day. But I was really pleased with how fast we had gotten up that 500 feet, and so after that Sungdare had an extra pair of gloves, and I had an extra pair too so we weren't too worried, and we just started sailing. We each had one bottle of oxygen, which I guess lasts about 7 hours with a Hornbein, and that's about what it did last, come to think of it.

"We just started moving like crazy up that middle gully you can see on the picture. Pretty soon I saw this blue—it looked like a tent—on the horizon. I thought, oh man, that's the Chinese east facers, you know. [Kop was referring to the American expedition tackling the Kangshung face on the east side of Everest; though he did not know it they had abandoned the mountain some days before.] It looked like a tent sticking there. It was about 800 feet above us. We really didn't stop because we only had a quart of water between us, and Sungdare didn't take any food. I took two little candy bars. You could see these little remnants of color up there where all the expeditions set their high camp. [Kop was referring to the old Camp 6 site at an altitude of about 8,400 meters (27,600 feet), which was used by, among others, the 1976 American Bicentennial expedition.] This blue object, the closer we got, I couldn't figure out what it was. And then we got quite close, and I realized it was a body— Hannelore Schmatz. We went right up this gully, and she was right there as we angled out from our camp, and you could see it from here—where Sungdare lost his gloves and he stashed a bottle of oxygen. [Kop is pointing to the sites on a photograph.] Helen was right there, and these other tents were right there, and I almost felt like waving because I thought this was the camp of the east face guys."

Hannelore Schmatz, German, and Ray Genet, American, were members of the 1979 German Everest expedition led by Gerhard Schmatz, Hannelore's husband. Hannelore and Genet reached the summit of Everest shortly after midday on October 2. The weather then deteriorated, and Schmatz, Genet, and Sungdare bivouacked at about 8,400 meters (27,600 feet). In the morning Genet was dead. Schmatz and Sungdare began the descent, and several sherpas came up from the South Col to help. However, when they reached Sungdare he told them that Hannelore Schmatz had collapsed and died shortly before. Sungdare himself was in critical condition and lost most of his toes. Now he was revisiting this place.

The Nepalese authorities had told us that the body of Hannelore Schmatz was on the route, and they had asked us to try to recover it. However, the body lies on a windswept icy section, and so it was impossible for Kop and Sungdare, or our subsequent climbers who saw the body, to bury it or evacuate it. This would require a group of people to go up from the Col with this specific objective. It is a considerable undertaking.* The body of Genet was not seen.

Kop continued: "Then we got up here, and I looked at my watch and I thought the watch had stopped because I just couldn't believe that we'd climbed that in an hour, an hour and twenty minutes, or something. I just refused to believe it. Actually what had happened is both our adrenalines were spurting so bad. On the way down I had the worst stomach problems—cramps in my leg, you know from the adrenaline spurts—I've ever experienced, and Sungdare kind of had the same thing.

"We continued on this ridge, which was very easy climbing, but right here there were some real dangerous wind slabs, and you had to get on the east face, and you hit your axe and you made a 'bonk' like that. We gingerly made our way up those wind slabs along the righthand side, and then you could see

---

*In 1984 two Nepalese climbers attempted to recover the body and both died in the attempt. One was Yogendra Thapa, our liaison officer.

the South Summit all the time. There was no wind from here up to the South Summit. Then we got near the South Summit, and we started getting the blasts again, you know, quite more powerful than the Col—about maybe 75 miles an hour. On the South Summit itself it was just a steady . . . you could lean into it kind of.

"And then the final ridge, in real life. I was scared. That final ridge is a pretty steep climb. If you slip there's really not much chance, so we belayed, boot-axe belayed each other, and I was really surprised—Sungdare really knows his stuff. He's really cautious, and he really knows how to do the standard belays, and he really cut himself a good platform, and we went faster than I expected. I was really happy when I saw him belaying me, you know, on these things.

"Then the Hillary Step . . . at that point I don't know what I was thinking, but I just went at it and tried to get at it the way Hillary did between the ice and rock, but it was so loose and so powdery in there that I couldn't get any firm footholds on the snow. I was afraid the whole thing was going to fall off the east face—it's just an overhanging cornice hooked onto the rock. It's about 70 degrees or so. And then I tried going right up on the rock and the ice, and then nearly slipped and fell there, and came down and breathed for five minutes as hard as I could. So then I went off to the left directly 90 degrees horizontal, and got onto the rock. The rock is fairly stratified horizontally to where you can get your crampon front points onto it, and then cut the ice off and work your way up that way.

"When I got to the top—I don't know how much time I spent breathing, but I was so scared, so wiped after getting to the top of that little 40 foot ridge—I just laid there, and Sungdare was yelling at me to get him up there. I checked my thing [oxygen set] and it was on 3, and I tried more oxygen— I just thought my lungs were going to burst. After he got up there it was . . . it's a series of very steep . . . you have to make your way left around on the southwest face—hummocks of ice, actually ice and real windpacked snow, and we just pumped our way. Then I could just see this little ridge like this right on the horizon, and I couldn't see any more hummocks beyond it, but I wasn't going to take the chance and find out there wasn't.

"So I just climbed over, and all of a sudden, damn, I was looking right down the north face, and I was looking down the east face, and I was standing right on the summit! I just jumped up and held my axe up, and Sungdare was throwing his arms around and . . . oh, shoot! We didn't have much to say to each other. I thought I was going to cry and everything else. I just said, man, don't cry here, your glasses will just get wiped out. I just wiped my glasses off, and couldn't do anything, so I whipped out my . . . the neatest picture—

101

everybody is going to get a picture of this. I've never seen a guy so proud in all my life. The first thing when Sungdare gets to the summit, he gets his Nepal flag out and he ties it to his axe and he stands up there with his chest out about that far—just like Tenzing. Oh, it was just a classic. Then I was going to try to show him how to take a picture of me. I just pulled out these little flags I had of Spokane, and put them on his chest. It was the most beautiful summit day, except for the wind, that you ever hope to have in the mountains.

"You could see Annapurna, Dhaulagiri, the Himalayas this way, and then Kangchenjunga, and Jannu, and Makalu was just chiseled—the peak that sticks out there. And then there wasn't a cloud through Tibet. You could see all those little just brown hills with a little white fang, a little tooth sticking out of it. You know, they are probably 20,000-foot peaks, but it's much warmer there, I guess. I don't know. Just brown hills . . . I just memorized the scene. I took some pictures in a series like this to prove that we were actually there . . . you know, you can triangulate it or whatever you want to do. The tripod wasn't there [Kop is referring to the tripod left on the summit by the 1975 Chinese expedition]. It was buried, we couldn't find it anywhere. Then the film started . . . it was cracking or something, and I would get so cold, probably it was 40 below and real hard winds. . . . So I stuck the camera back in my shirt, and it warmed up and I took more shots on the way down."

A VOICE: It didn't tear?

KOP: I hope not. I probably took six or eight of Sungdare with his chest stuck out a mile. He was . . . that was his moment, boy.

ANOTHER VOICE: You took some of Tibet . . .

KOP: Yeah, I did take one looking down the north ridge, and I was really surprised at the steepness of it, you know. You know, it always looks in the pictures. Everest looks like this big hump. Boy, it's a mountain. It's got its technical points like every other one.

ANOTHER VOICE: But there was plenty of room on top for both of you, on the summit?

KOP: Yeah, it's a ridge, maybe 50 to 75 feet long that's the same elevation, and it comes off the west ridge, and then the east face is here. It looked like a kind of cornice area that was actually the same height, but

I didn't want to step on it. We were definitely on the summit. There was nowhere else to go. We probably didn't spend half an hour, maybe 20 minutes, because you start getting cold in that wind, start moving again.

ANOTHER VOICE: Did you rappel the Step going down? [The reference is to the Hillary Step, which is a difficult pitch between the main summit and south summit.]

KOP: No. I played a big chicken move there. I asked Sungdare if he would belay me down the ridge, and I would try to find a better way down—not on the rock, on the overhanging . . . the snow. Because it looked like you could climb . . . you know where Doug Scott [actually Kop is referring to a photograph of Dougal Haston climbing the Hillary Step; it was taken by Doug Scott] . . . you've seen that picture of him climbing . . . and I thought I could chop a real good spot down there. Well, it turned out that it was just sugary, and I got down and he had me on tension. So I went into the rock, and I made a good step into the snow and a good step on the rock, and a good step in the snow and a good one on the rock . . . back and forth. Then I got to the bottom, and I cut myself a real good belay spot because if he did take a fall he would go right down in the snow.

Well, he tried that and the thing I didn't think about is my legs are quite a bit longer than his. He came down a couple of steps, and then went back up, and then climbed down the rock the way we went up. It took him about 10 or 15 minutes, but he made every move down. You know, there's quite a few Hillary Steps up there. I'm serious. You go out of the . . . you come right out of the South Summit, and you've got a real steep section of . . . I guess it just depends on how you hit it, you know. It changes every season I'm sure. But Sungdare said it was far more dangerous than when he went in 1979. . . .

You know what's really amazing about these sherpas, their strength and their training, what they grow up with. In the morning I said, "Sungdare, I only

103

have one quart of liquid for all day." He says, ". . . no necessary for me. Maybe just a little." And he did— maybe an inch out of that quart, that's all he wanted at the South Summit. But he's really quite incredible. I don't know what it is. Metabolism? Control and whatnot that they have. He didn't eat anything. He had . . . I offered him some Grandma's cookies, but I had about half of them.

EVANS: At what point did you realize or really feel like you were going to make it?

KOP: Oh, about 50 yards from the summit. It's really touch and go all the way because I was . . . when you climb with someone you've never climbed with before every- thing is in your own head, you know. You're not . . . I don't look back on the rope, and think, well, if I can't lead this he can. It's always boy can I lead the next one, or can I keep leading these things, or can I keep kicking steps. And when I saw the summit ridge, maybe that was the lack of emotion. I was so beat out when I kicked up over the top, and said, hey here we are, great, for God's sake don't cry. But I really didn't feel confident till just the very . . . till actually seeing that there were no hummocks after the last skyline. And as fast as we were going, as strong as Sungdare is, you still need . . . you know, it's almost like we were soloing the thing in our minds.

ANOTHER VOICE: Did it take you very long to get down?

KOP: Oh, I think maybe three hours. We ran out of oxygen down in those gullies. Sungdare had not . . . that was another interesting thing. I had burned up maybe an hour and a half faster on the same liter-per-minute setting of oxygen than he had. I just couldn't believe my eyes.

ANOTHER VOICE: You were on setting 3 most of the time?

KOP: Yeah, I went on 3 all the way. And I saw that old camp over there, and Sungdare went over and got a

Luxfer bottle. It's about 20 feet from where we were having a little snack. It was just dead calm. On the way down we were sitting on this shoulder, 27,500 feet, and it was just like we were sitting in the Canadian Rockies with your wife and kids, you know, on the tailgate of the car. Really, there was no wind or nothing. We were having a snack and shooting the breeze, and I said, "I wonder if there is any oxygen in that." He says, "Oh, I'll go look and see." And he brought a bottle. It was only 100 feet away and it was 2,000 PSI, it was '76 Bicentennial oxygen. It was really amazing.

ANOTHER VOICE: Did you use that bottle?

KOP: Yeah, I went down. I still can't believe it happened the way it did. Because I was ready to just say we'll take . . . we were planning on taking just oxygen up for the next group, because it was so windy. And it just turned out lucky. That day was just . . . as Sungdare said, we were very lucky.

ANOTHER VOICE: Did you say you saw both bodies?

KOP: No, no, I did say that Sungdare said this is where Genet died. And, I don't know, I had the spookiest . . .

ANOTHER VOICE: But the woman's body was in the same spot?

KOP: No, the woman was down further. She started down very slowly, and ran out of oxygen and died immediately I guess, according to Sungdare. I made a burial—you know, some little religious things that you do, you know my own personal feelings towards these people. You know . . . Genet. . . .

ANOTHER VOICE: Did you know him?

KOP: Yeah, I knew him pretty well. He helped a friend of mine out on Mount McKinley. I conversed with him for about a week during a storm up there, and got to know his psyche and whatnot pretty well. It was really. . . . I think it was obviously just that I had these really strong feelings that here was this guy that I knew laying there dead, you know. I couldn't get it out of my mind.

ANOTHER VOICE: But did you actually see . . . ?

KOP: No, no. I didn't see him. Sungdare pointed out the spot where he dug the hole, and Genet was laying there. And Sungdare says he's not here—obviously blown away or fallen down the mountain or something. But he showed me all the exact spots, you know, and the woman's body was just 100 yards down below.

ANOTHER VOICE: Did you just stop at Camp 5 long enough to pack up your stuff?

KOP: Yeah, we came back to Camp 5, and it was blowing like crazy. Same old winds. And I was going to try . . . I was thinking all the way down I wanted to do. I was thinking of you, John, all the way. I wanted to do a bicycle thing to see what I could do. [Kop is referring to a measurement of maximal exercise on the stationary bicycle that had been taken up to Camp 5.] But I had these horrendous stomach cramps that I just couldn't get rid of. So we just grabbed our bags, and headed on down to 4. When we got to 4 we found out there was no sleeping there, so we went to 3. I piled up oxygen all around the Camp 5 settlement so it would protect that tent from the wind as much as possible. Then we stuck an extra Ensolite [foam pad] inside to make it kind of a little igloo, you know, so when C-sahib [nickname for Pizzo] and Peter go up they have at least a shelter there.

ANOTHER VOICE: How many full bottles were there at 5?

KOP: Oh, it was about eight. We just used two full bottles. Seven or eight I should say.

ANOTHER VOICE: Both you and Sungdare went on oxygen then as you went up?

KOP: Yeah, we went full bore as much as the body would take. It definitely keeps your mind alert. I took the mask off on the summit and on the South Summit, but that's kind of a shock to the system—boy, it's pretty thin up there. I mean, you start getting numb . . .

EVANS: Did you have a chance to fill in C-sahib and Hackett?

KOP: I spent about an hour and a half. Yeah, C-sahib, I told him exactly where I laid everything, and put all the food in the tent, and had all the oxygen . . . the full ones on this side, and the empty ones on this side. I think that maybe he and Young Tenzing and Hackett might try to get rigged up and go, because C-sahib is a real gambler. I told him once you get around those gullies . . . I really hope that they do.

EVANS: When you left Camp 5 was the wind coming up out of the Cwm here?

KOP: It comes right over the Cwm, and sweeps over there, that's the way it was that day. And then at the South Summit there was that jet-stream effect. It was probably, I would say at least 60-mile-an-hour winds, maybe 70, 75, steady, on the summit ridge. But at that point you go beyond thinking rationally, and you just keep going. The wind was coming right up the west ridge. It was just so clear, not a speck of dust, you know, and then India was all a layer of clouds, and then the clouds came up into the foothills of Nepal. Thyangboche was down there, you could see that, and Pheriche, all those towns. Sungdare was pointing out all those little towns. And then on the other side I was trying to look for Lhasa, but I think it is about 100 miles away. But I was looking for little signs of life in the brown hills there.

ANOTHER VOICE: Did you leave anything on top?

KOP: No. I was going to leave these little flags that I had tied to the tripod, but the tripod wasn't there so I took them out and showed them the summit and put them back in.

ANOTHER VOICE: What flags did you have on top?

KOP: Unfortunately, I just had a Spokane mountaineer emblem.

ANOTHER VOICE: That's going ato look bad.

ANOTHER VOICE: He's a local guy (laughter).

KOP: Oh, I don't care about that stuff anyway. I should have had an AMREE flag or something. Do we have any of those? I couldn't believe Sungdare. He was prepared. I mean, he just got to the summit and he points to me like this—take my picture—and he ties the flag from the tip to the top [of his ice axe], and his legs are all spread out . . . You wait till you see it. I hope they came out. Yeah, he's a real nice guy, too, a real gentleman.

ANOTHER VOICE: He's a little bit richer than he was before he went up there, too, isn't he? 500 rupees.

KOP: No, I changed that. I changed that to 1,000 rupees. What the hell is 100 bucks? Yeah, and he didn't seem to bat an eye. But I said, look, Sungdare, it's very important to this expedition that some sahib gets up there. I said I was going to pay Annu 500 rupees, but he got sick. He could have had the whole works, 1,000 rupees. But still he's got the sense to know that money, you know, is not worth it . . . plus I said I'd give him my jacket, my watch. I felt like I was doing something wrong by that, you know, for a little bit, but what the heck. This is . . . we're not going to be here again. This is it.

ANOTHER VOICE: The expedition would be willing to pay that 1,000 rupees.

KOP: No, that's my deal between him and me. Don't worry about that. The expedition's got nothing to pay. That was a private enterprise deal.

The news of Kop and Sungdare's success reached us at Camp 2 at about 4 P.M. Sungdare was the first to reach Camp 3, and he radioed the news down to the sherpas at 2. Sonam burst into the laboratory with his hands in the air, shouting, "success!" and naturally the elation was terrific. Many of us had despaired of the expedition reaching the summit after the disappointments of the last couple of weeks, and the ferocious weather at Camp 5.

Kop and Sungdare came down to Camp 2 the following morning. There is all the difference in the world between an expedition that gets to the summit, and one that does not, even though we still needed additional scientific data at extreme altitudes. We had a long debriefing session, and recorded Kop's account. Kop presented various expedition members with small rocks from near the summit.

Kop was the ninth American to set foot on the summit of Mt. Everest. Five members of the first American expedition in 1963 reached the summit: Jim Whittaker, Barry Bishop, and Lute Jerstad from the South Col, and Tom Hornbein and Willi Unsoeld via the West Ridge. The latter two made the first ascent by this route, and then completed the traverse descending via the South Col. Two climbers reached the summit during the 1976 Bicentennial Expedition—Chris Chandler and Bob Cormack. (Chris helped with preparations for our expedition. He wore one of our Medilog recorders to the summit, and obtained a successful electrocardiogram up to an altitude of about 7,300 meters [24,000 feet].) Finally, Ray Genet, a member of the 1979 German expedition, reached the summit via the South Col route.

Needless to say, all the climbers and climbing scientists share the credit for the summit achievement. John Evans particularly had good reason to be satisfied. His many years of planning had paid off, and in spite of his personal disappointment at not being able to get to the highest camps, he never lost control of the situation, and his solid leadership was evident all the way.

Even though Kop and Sungdare were not able to do any science at the summit, reaching the top of Mt. Everest is no small triumph, and it certainly made all the difference to our expedition. There was a big psychological impact—a realization that although conditions at Camp 5 might be appallingly bad, above that altitude the wind would be tolerable. The Hillary Step was difficult but was passable. Kop and Sungdare cut steps, and the next climbers could make use of them. A barrier had been broken. However, it was now essential for us to get some scientific data above Camp 5, and this brings us to the next chapter.

8
SCIENCE ON TOP

"It was written in the wind"[1]

When Chris Pizzo and Peter Hackett set out from Camp 2 for Camp 4 early on the morning of October 21, most of the remaining climbers and climbing scientists were not fit enough to make a summit attempt. Of course, Chris Kopczynski was in the process of doing just that with sherpa Sungdare. But most of the other climbers had recently been up to Camp 5 in appalling weather conditions, and they needed some respite. Davey Jones had come down from Camp 5 on the 14th looking exhausted from the gale force winds; he was well below par. Glenn Porzak was still suffering from his ordeal at Camp 5; he had lost almost all his voice. Jeff Lowe had developed early high-altitude pulmonary edema; his face had a distinctly blueish coloration indicating that his lungs were not doing a good job of oxygenating the blood.

The climbing scientists were also showing signs of wear and tear. Steve Boyer had evidence of pulmonary edema, and used oxygen for sleeping on the night of the 20th. Both Dave Graber and Frank Sarnquist had done a great job carrying to 5, but they were not anxious to go up again. Brownie Schoene was not happy above Camp 3, probably because of his low ventilatory response to hypoxia as discussed in Chapter 6.

So it seemed that if we were to obtain scientific measurements above Camp

5, our hopes rested on Chris and Peter. And even they were not in the best condition. Peter had severe bronchitis with a hacking cough when he left Camp 2. Chris had been inactive at Camp 2 for a week, and was just not feeling his best. We all had our fingers crossed when they set out on the 21st for Camp 3.

Pizzo takes up the story on the tape that he recorded when he eventually returned to Camp 2. "Well, I got up to the headwall, and started zooming. I got up to Camp 4 without oxygen in 6 or 7 hours. Peter was slower; he was definitely weak. He was feeling his physical ailments, but he got up there okay, and then as it turned out we had an enforced rest day at 4, which was probably a blessing in disguise."

This rest day was a result of one of those accidents that can happen so easily at extreme altitudes. One of the sherpas was passing a stove to another tent, and lost control of it; it was last seen tumbling down the slope of the headwall heading for the Cwm 1,200 meters (4,000 feet) below! Because they had no spare stove, another had to be brought up from Camp 3, and this cost a day. Meanwhile, the weather was good, and everyone at Camp 2 was biting his nails fearing that a chance for a summit attempt had been missed.

Living conditions at camps 3 and 4 were extremely difficult at this time. Both camps were extremely tight for space because there was no level area outside the platforms. Several tents had been damaged by storms. Hygiene was bad; it was not easy to find uncontaminated ice to melt for drinking water. Mike Weis and Jeff Lowe were particularly bitter about the conditions at 3 and 4 when they arrived back at Camp 2 on October 21.

Chris continues. "Next day [October 23] I woke up and felt great again, and I zoomed up to 5, passing two sherpas. Peter did moderately well, and when I met him up there he said, 'yeah, maybe I'll think about going for the summit too.'

"And then it got very complicated talking to Nuru Jangbo who didn't really know if he wanted to go or not, and should we do a four-man rope team or a three-man rope team, etc., etc., and finally we decided on the two rope teams." The first of these would be Chris Pizzo and Young Tenzing, and the second Peter Hackett and Nuru Jangbo.

When they got to Camp 5 Chris and Peter dug out the scientific equipment, which had been buried in one of the tents, and set everything up for the summit bid the following morning. (Peter knew where the equipment was, unlike Kop three days before, because he had repacked it after his previous climb to Camp 5.) They put on the special vests with electrodes for recording the electrocardiogram. The electrodes themselves were taped onto the chest, one on the top of the breast bone in front, and one on each side of the chest halfway down.

A special pocket in the vest contained the Medilog recorder, a slow-running four-channel tape recorder that was turned on when they left Camp 5 in the morning, and turned off when they returned in the evening. In this way physiological information could be collected all day long without any intervention by the climber. The Medilog recorder would be near the skin of the climber, and therefore kept warm by his body. Thus the intricate mechanism would not freeze and stop.

In addition to the electrocardiogram, the Medilog recorder had a timing channel to indicate elapsed time on the tape so that the time of day of a particular recorded event could be determined. The climbers made a note of the time the recorder was turned on. There was also an event marker with four different colored buttons; the climber kept this in the pocket of his jacket. When a button was pressed it encoded a signal on the tape, which assisted in its interpretation later.

Finally, there was a small flow meter attached to a mouthpiece for measuring the amount of air that was breathed. To use this, the climber took off his oxygen gear, and climbed for several minutes breathing through the flow meter. A small turbine inside spun as the air passed over it, and this interrupted a beam of light that placed pulses on the slow-running tape. We were thus able to determine the amount of air going in and out of the lungs (ventilation) during hard climbing.

Pizzo also packed one of the alveolar gas samplers, a special piece of equipment for taking samples of air from the depths of the lungs. The climber put his lips around the mouthpiece and exhaled fully. Special valves ensured that the last exhaled gas from the deepest parts of the lungs remained in the sample chamber of the instrument. The climber then pulled a lever that opened the valve of a small aluminum can inside the sampler. This can had been evacuated in San Diego so that when the valve was opened, air from the sampling chamber was sucked into it. When the lever was released the valve closed, thus trapping the gas; and at the same time the cartridge holding the cans rotated to bring another aluminum can into the sampling position. The climber could take six samples of alveolar gas with no other maneuvers than breathing out fully and pulling the lever six times.

The preevacuated aluminum cans were transported from UC San Diego to Camp 5 in strong glass tubes that were also evacuated. This reduced the danger of any air leaking in during the long trip. One of the jobs Chris had to do on the afternoon of the 23rd when he was preparing for his summit bid was to take the aluminum cans out of their protective glass tubes and insert them into the cartridges in preparation for taking the alveolar gas samples.

Chris also carried a small dictating tape recorder, which he kept in the inside pocket of his down jacket. He recorded comments about what he was doing at various times so that we could interpret the Medilog tapes later. It also provided a dramatic commentary on his summit climb.

He also put the barometer-thermometer in his backpack in preparation for measurements of barometric pressure and temperature as high as possible. This ingenious device had been designed by Karl Maret using a highly accurate crystal sensor lent to us by Airesearch Corporation in California. The climber had simply to depress a button, and the barometric pressure was accurately displayed in large numbers on the dial—a jumbo version of the liquid crystal display used in modern digital watches. When he pressed a second button the barometric pressure was replaced by temperature. One of the most important functions of the tape recorder was to enable the climber to immediately record his observation of pressure and temperature. As a backup in case something happened to the tape recorder, Chris carried photographs of the route from the South Col to the summit. He could mark his position on the photograph, and indicate the pressure and temperature by checking boxes with a grease pencil. In the event, it was not necessary to use these cards because the dictating recorder worked so well.

Chris takes up the story on his pocket recorder. "This is C-sahib at Camp 5 on the 24th of October, or whatever it is. I turned on my Medilog at 5 o'clock. It is now about 6:20. We're about 10 minutes away from taking off. I just pushed event marker 1. The barometric pressure at Camp 5 at this time is 284.5. [The pressure was recorded in millimeters of mercury.]"

The next recording was made almost three hours later. "It's 9 o'clock. I figure I'm about two-thirds or three-quarters of the way to the South Summit, about 150 vertical feet below Camp 6. It's 9 o'clock (did I say that already?). I just pushed the white event marker. The barometric pressure is 271.4, temperature 5.8 [centigrade], make that negative 5.8. It's a spectacular day. There are low clouds in the valleys and plains. I can see over the Nuptse ridge now to Thyangboche. Makalu is spectacular. I'm about three-quarters of the way up. . . . We've been a little slower than I thought, but still on schedule. I've used a little less than half a tank of gas."

At about this time one of those almost miraculous events occurred, one that had a profound effect on the outcome of our expedition. To backtrack for a moment, Chris along with Kop and Davey had established Camp 5 on October 11, and when it was time to go down on the 14th because of the impossible weather, Chris had left his ice axe at 5. This was reasonable because there was a fixed rope all the way from 5 down to the Cwm, and there was no point in carrying unnecessary weight. However, during the nine days he was away from Camp 5, there had been terrific storms, and when he tried to find his ice axe on the afternoon of the 23rd it was nowhere to be seen. It was in fact there, but now buried under snow and ice.

This left Chris in a quandary. There was no spare ice axe at 5. However, he was reluctant to postpone the summit attempt in what appeared to be reasonable weather, particularly as the end of October was approaching, and conditions were likely to deteriorate. He set off on the morning of October 24 using the best substitute he could find for an ice axe—a tent pole!

There is no way that you can get to the summit of Mt. Everest with a tent pole. The final summit ridge is sufficiently steep, and the snow conditions there are sufficiently treacherous, that an ice axe is essential for safety. Imagine Chris's astonishment when about 30 meters (100 feet) below the old Camp 6 site he came across a "beautiful titanium-steel ice axe" sticking up out of the snow in the middle of his path, just like the sword Excalibur! As Chris said afterward, "I then knew I would make the summit—it was written in the wind!"

We subsequently found out that this was the ice axe that Hannelore Schmatz had been using in October 1979. It had been rattling around Mt. Everest for two years, and turned up exposed on the ice right in front of Chris just when he needed it. This near miracle not only allowed Chris to get to the summit; it was responsible for us obtaining the critical scientific measurements on the summit. If ever proof were needed of the high lama of Thyangboche's assertion that luck was the most important element for success, this was it!

Incidentally, this ice axe has now been to the summit three times. Gerhard Schmatz, the leader of the 1979 expedition, took it with him to the summit and then gave it to his wife for her successful climb after he had returned to the South Col. An interesting question is who is the rightful owner of the ice axe—this was raised by Herr Schmatz in some correspondence after the expedition. I decided to leave the resolution of that knotty one to Schmatz and Pizzo.

Shortly after this, Chris made a measurement of maximal exercise ventilation while climbing. He took off his oxygen, breathed through the flow meter, and climbed as hard as he could for about 7 minutes. (The recording on the Medilog tape was technically excellent.) His average ventilation was about 107 liters per minute, considerably less than his maximum ventilation at Camp 2, because the amount of work he was able to do at an altitude of 8,300 meters (27,200 feet) was very much less. The recording showed that he was breathing at the extremely rapid rate of 86 breaths per minute—fast but shallowly. His maximum heart rate was about 134 beats per minute, which as in the case of his ventilation, was considerably less than the maximal value at lower altitudes. Again this was mainly because he was not able to work as hard at this oxygen-deprived altitude.

Chris's comments on the tape recorder were brief and to the point. "I've done spirometry from 9:20 to 9:25. Start with green event marker, stop with red event marker. I've covered about 25 vertical feet, and it was a bitch. I'm going back on oxygen. See you later."

Chris found the wind conditions from Camp 5 to the South Summit much as Kop described. About half an hour after he and Young Tenzing turned the corner and got into the gully, there was almost no wind. It was only when they reached the South Summit that they encountered the high winds, and these persisted right up to the summit. He said on the debriefing tape when he returned to Camp 2: "There's really an interesting contrast. We've been fooled by the Camp 5 situation this whole time. It's constantly windy there—that's the natural gully where the wind is going. About half an hour around the corner there's no wind. Even when you hit the summit ridge there's no wind till you get to the South Summit. And then at the South Summit you encounter the same wind that's on the Col—west to east. And most of the day I was overdressed. I was sweating like hell. I was peeling clothes off. Then I got to the South Summit, and started putting them back on again. It wasn't that bad. We were lucky. We had definitely good conditions.

"I was surprised at the technical difficulties between the South Summit and true summit. It's essentially a knife edge ridge, and the Hillary Step is halfway in between. There's 15 feet of vertical crud—mixed rock and snow—and I'll tell you what; it really wasn't that bad yesterday because of Kop's and Sungdare's steps, although I did a slight variation of their route in the Hillary Step. Still, that whole summit ridge was a lot safer because of their steps. We stepped in their steps, and they were firm. Outside the steps it was soft; you would sink in, and it was unstable. It really eased the technical difficulties incredibly. Young Tenzing was very iffy the whole time, very worried, always asking me how much longer it was going to take to the South Summit, and when we got to the South Summit the wind started blowing, and he started complaining. I led everything, and all the good he did me was to belay me on the Hillary Step. And he did set up a good ice axe belay."

Chris and Young Tenzing reached the summit at 12:30 P.M. On the tape the summit wind sounds like a passing jet aircraft, and Chris is clearly extremely short of breath. Yet the excitement and enthusiasm come through as he pants his exultant message into the recorder.

"Okay. I think it's working. The time is 12:30. Young Tenzing and I just made the summit! The barometric pressure is 253.0, repeat 253.0. The temperature inside my pack was −8.8. It's a beautiful clear day. There are some clouds in the valley and lowlands. As soon as we hit the summit there became very high winds. It's cold right now. I don't think we will stick around too long. Been here about 15 minutes. I'm going to try to take some alveolar gas samples and do a spirometry, but I'll report back later. Over."

Chris and Young Tenzing spent half an hour on the summit, and Chris accomplished a tremendous amount. First he took a series of photographs including a fine one of Young Tenzing holding his ice axe in the air. He then took out a Frisbee, which he threw off in the direction of the east face because the wind was blowing from west to east. As Chris said later, "it wasn't my greatest throw, but it did disappear from sight somewhere down in the east basin, and eventually boomeranged back into the mountain as all Frisbees do if you throw them off at a high enough point, and there was a wind to throw it off center."

Next Chris measured the barometric pressure and temperature. The barometric pressure of 253 was a little higher than we expected, partly because there was a high-pressure weather system at the time. The temperature of minus 8.8 degrees indicates that Chris and Young Tenzing had an exceptionally fine day.

Finally, Chris prepared to take the alveolar gas samples. First he took the sampler out of his backpack and attached one of the cartridges. Then he took off his oxygen mask and set up for the photograph shown in the photo insert. This was taken with Chris actually sitting on the summit.

Young Tenzing has been holding the camera while Chris was preparing the alveolar gas sampler and according to Chris "he took a couple of very strange pictures of his pack and his ice axe at close range that were out of focus, I think." So Chris took the camera, set up the proper exposure and focus, and gave it to Young Tenzing to take the shot. The first thing the sherpa did was to start twisting all the dials around and naturally Chris expected the worst. However, as can be seen, the photograph was perfect—you can even read the expedition logo on the alveolar gas sampler. Also, the exposure was superb, a very difficult feat in the conditions of intense light on the summit. Young Tenzing was clearly a better photographer than we gave him credit for!

After the photograph was taken, Chris set to work taking the alveolar gas samples. Here he encountered an unexpected problem—the cartridge on the sampler would not rotate properly, probably because of the intense cold. So Chris had to put the individual ampules in to the cartridge one by one. He later reported: "It was hard. Those fourth, fifth, and sixth ones were really hard, and I remember the exhalation would . . . from blowing out the last bit . . . was making me a little dizzy. . . . Also, during the last three samples was when Young Tenzing started getting restless, and was begging me to get out of there because even though it was a beautiful day, the winds were blowing up there and it was cold, and my hands were numb. As soon as I took my mittens off exposing my gloved hands, my fingers were numb."

117

Chris insisted that as long as he was sitting still on the summit without oxygen, he felt fine. "There was no discomfort whatsoever. But the slightest movement, the slightest activity where I really had to move my entire body from one place to another would make a drastic difference, and a really marked increase in ventilation."

Chris and Young Tenzing started down from the summit as soon as the alveolar gas collection had been completed. This was none too soon for the sherpa. Back at Camp 2 Chris described negotiating the Hillary Step. "Down climbing the Hillary Step was not too much fun. I didn't take a step without making sure I was well oxygenated. Not the place where you want to make a mistake, even on belay. Peter fell there on the way down. He was extremely lucky. You don't want to fall there or you'll come right down this [southwest] face. . . . You're on this side of the ridge all the way. As a matter of fact, from the South Summit to the Hillary Step, which is about half, two-thirds of the way to the summit, you can look right down to Camp 2. A good set of binoculars here would have sighted the climbers."

The two climbers were just below the South Summit when to their surprise they met Peter Hackett. He was alone because his companion, Nuru Jangbo, had become too cold to continue, and had therefore returned to Camp 5. Chris and Peter discussed the situation, and thereby hangs a tale that will be taken up in the next chapter.

What is the significance of the measurements made at Camp 5 and above, including the summit? Some of the most interesting results came from the alveolar gas data. In all, 42 samples were obtained at 8,050 meters (26,200 feet) and above, including 6 samples on the summit. I personally carried the samples back to UC San Diego in a special box and they were analyzed in our laboratory using a mass spectrometer. Eight ampules were empty or contained ambient air, and so did not provide useful data. The results of the remainder were fascinating.

The most striking finding was the extremely low level of carbon dioxide pressure in the lungs on the summit. Figure 6 shows the means of the data collected by Pizzo, and measurements made by previous expeditions at barometric pressures below 350 millimeters of mercury. All the data are from lowlanders acclimatized to high altitudes. Note that although there is considerable scatter in the measurements, the partial pressure of carbon dioxide (Pco_2) falls to about 7.5 millimeters of mercury on the summit. The normal value at sea level is 40. This reduction reflects the increase in ventilation (volume of each breath times breathing rate) in climbers at these extreme altitudes.

The fall in Pco_2 was considerably more than we had predicted. On the

118

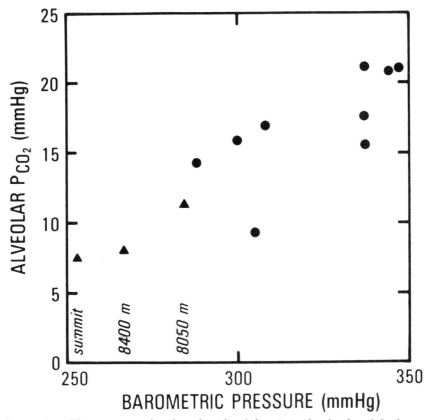

Figure 6. The pressure of carbon dioxide of the air in the depths of the lungs (alveolar Pco_2) plotted against barometric pressure, which decreases as altitude increases. Triangles show the means of results found on this expedition; circles refer to previous expeditions.

basis of measurements made at somewhat lower altitudes, I thought the most likely Pco_2 on the summit would be about 10 millimeters of mercury. Although the measured value of 7.5 may not seem much lower, that 2.5 millimeters of mercury makes a world of difference at these altitudes.

The advantage of the high ventilation at these altitudes is that it tends to maintain or "defend" the partial pressure of oxygen (Po_2) in the lungs. This is apparent in Figure 7. Note that as altitude increases we follow the curve down from top right to bottom left. Both the alveolar Pco_2 and Po_2 decrease as subjects ascend higher. The Pco_2 falls because of the increasing ventilation, and the Po_2 falls because the inspired oxygen is reduced.

Note, however, that at Pco_2 values below about 15 (corresponding to altitudes above about 7,000 meters or 23,000 feet) there is no further fall in P_{O_2}. Instead it is maintained or "defended" at a level of about 35 millimeters of mercury in spite of the fact that the inspired P_{O_2} is falling because of the decrease in barometric pressure. This is clearly advantageous to the body because it insulates, as it were, the body from the progressively falling inspired P_{O_2}.

This tremendous hyperventilation is probably one of the most important mechanisms of acclimatization to these extreme altitudes. However, as we saw in Chapter 6 when the other scientific measurements were being discussed, there is considerable variability among individuals in their ability to respond to high altitude by hyperventilating. Not everybody can mount the increased degree of ventilation necessary for defending the alveolar P_{O_2} as shown in Figure 7. This may well explain why there is such a good correlation between

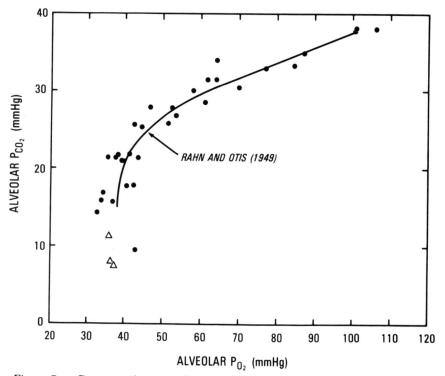

Figure 7. Pressure of oxygen (horizontal axis) and pressure of carbon dioxide (vertical axis) in the air from the depths of the lungs as subjects are acclimatized to higher and higher altitudes. (Our measurements are triangles; circles are results from previous studies.) Sea level is top right, and the summit of Mt. Everest is bottom left.

120

hypoxic ventilatory response and tolerance to extreme altitude, as we discussed in relation to Figure 5.

However, the P_{O_2} in the depths of the lungs (alveolar P_{O_2}) is only part of the story. The more important value to the climber is actually the P_{O_2} in the arterial blood distributed throughout the body. Unfortunately, it is impossible to take a sample of arterial blood on the summit with present technology. It was in fact a considerable tour de force for Pizzo to take samples of alveolar gas.

However, we can obtain some information about the arterial P_{O_2} by calculating the changes in oxygen as the blood moves through the capillaries of the lungs. Here a few words about the anatomy of the lungs may be useful. The blood is contained in capillaries, and is separated from the alveolar air in the lungs by an extremely thin membrane—less than one-thousandth of a millimeter thick. As the blood flows along the capillary, oxygen moves from the alveolar air across this thin barrier to the blood by a process of passive diffusion. That is, the oxygen flows from a region of relatively high partial pressure in the alveolar air to a region of low pressure in the blood rather as water flows downhill. As a consequence the P_{O_2} of the blood gradually rises along the capillary, and normally it reaches the alveolar value by the time the blood leaves the lungs.

This means that the oxygen pressure in the blood can never exceed the value in the alveolar gas. Since the latter is only 35 millimeters of mercury, the blood P_{O_2} must be extremely low. Of course, it would be even lower if the very high level of ventilation had not raised the alveolar P_{O_2} to 35.

The situation is even worse at extreme altitudes. It turns out that the rate at which oxygen can be loaded into the blood is much slower because of the low alveolar oxygen pressure. Partly as a result of this the P_{O_2} of the blood rises very slowly, and has nowhere near reached the alveolar value before the blood leaves the lungs. In other words, there is just not sufficient time for the normal transfer of oxygen to take place. The net result is that the P_{O_2} of the arterial blood never reaches even the alveolar value, which is itself extremely low.

Thus when we calculate the changes of oxygen occurring in the blood in the lungs of a climber on the summit using all the available data, we find that the arterial P_{O_2} is only about 28 millimeters of mercury. This is a desperately low value—it is rarely seen in even the most severe lung disease, and then usually indicates impending death. The normal value in healthy young people is nearly 100. The value of 28 graphically underlines the extraordinary oxygen deprivation within the body at these extreme altitudes.[2]

We were also able to calculate the acidity of Pizzo's blood on the summit because this is determined in part by the P_{CO_2} in the arterial blood (which is the same as that in alveolar gas). Here we used information obtained from blood samples collected by Chris and Peter Hackett on the morning of the 25th, the day after their summit climbs. The results showed that the pH of the arterial blood was over 7.7 (the normal sea level value is 7.4). Again this is an astonishingly abnormal value. The body usually jealously preserves the pH of the arterial blood within a very narrow range, and it is almost incredible that it would allow the pH to increase to this extent.

Interestingly enough, there is some evidence that this high blood pH is beneficial at high altitudes. The reason is technical. It seems that an increased pH speeds up the loading of oxygen by blood in the lungs. The mechanism has to do with the effect of pH on the binding of oxygen by hemoglobin—at a high pH the affinity of hemoglobin for oxygen is increased. At any event, this factor may partly explain the "deterioration" that rapidly occurs in climbers at extreme altitudes. It is well known that a climber who spends more than two or three days at 8,000 meters (26,200 feet) quickly loses condition. A possible reason is that the kidneys begin to restore the blood pH to nearer normal, and thus the advantage of the high pH on oxygen loading in the lungs is lost. However, it should be added that limited data from our expedition indicate that the kidney is changing blood pH very slowly at these altitudes, possibly because of dehydration of the body, so this explanation is no more than a hypothesis.

The combination of values for arterial P_{O_2}, P_{CO_2}, and pH of 28, 7.5, and over 7.7 respectively represent such a deranged situation that it is remarkable that a climber on the summit is even alive, let alone able to carry out simple tasks. These astonishing results confirm the contention made earlier, that man on the summit of Everest without supplementary oxygen must be at the limits of human tolerance.

Turning to barometric pressure, Pizzo measured 253 millimeters of mercury. As indicated earlier, this was about 3 millimeters higher than we had predicted, and the difference can probably be attributed mainly to the high-pressure weather conditions at the time. The exceptionally high temperature of about minus 9 degrees centigrade is consistent with this.

The relationship between barometric pressure and altitude on Mt. Everest is itself an interesting topic.[3] It was pointed out some years ago that the pressure found at a given altitude tends to be considerably higher than that predicted from the standard altitude-pressure tables. These tables are used by the aviation industry, and are employed by physiologists and physicians to predict the oxygen deprivation of man exposed to various altitudes.

The pressures that we measured from Base Camp to the summit were all indeed higher than the standard tables indicate (Figure 8). The measured pressure on the summit was 17 millimeters of mercury higher than the value in the standard tables. The reason is that barometric pressure at these altitudes depends very much on latitude. Near the equator the pressure is relatively high; near the poles it is lower. These differences in turn can be explained by radiation and convection currents.

There is a large mass of very cold air in the stratosphere above the equator. (Paradoxically, the coldest air in the atmosphere is above the equator.) Because this cold air is relatively heavy, it increases the pressure below it at altitudes of about 4 to 16 kilometers above the earth's surface, and this range includes the summits of the highest mountains.

An interesting corollary of all of this is that if Mr. Everest were situated at a higher latitude (for example, that of Mt. McKinley) it would be impossible

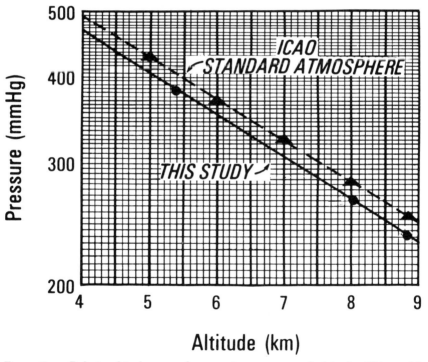

Figure 8.   Relationship between barometric pressure and altitude. This could be used to measure altitude on Everest in May or October if an accurate barometer were available.

for a climber to reach the summit without supplementary oxygen. In other words, this climatic idiosyncrasy makes it just possible for man to reach the highest point on earth breathing Mother Nature's air.

There are other interesting implications. We know from measurements made by meteorological balloons that barometric pressure at these altitudes varies by over 10 millimeters of mercury between summer and winter. A climber attempting to reach the summit of Mt. Everest without supplementary oxygen in January would be at a considerable disadvantage because of the low barometric pressure, quite apart from the obvious problems of cold and wind. Not surprisingly, a winter ascent without supplementary oxygen has not yet been successful.

Even the day-to-day variations of barometric pressure on the summit of Everest, which amount to 2–3 millimeters of mercury, may affect the amount of work a climber can do. This is because the work capacity of a climber under these conditions is exquisitely sensitive to small changes in barometric pressure. A climber at Camp 5 who plans an "oxygenless" ascent might want to consult his barometer first!

The results we obtained at altitudes over 8,000 meters (26,200 feet) throw considerable light on how man can tolerate these extreme altitudes. Prior to the expedition my colleague Dr. Peter Wagner and I carried out a theoretical study of the physiology of a climber on the summit. It was difficult for us to see how enough oxygen could be available to the body for a climber to reach the summit without using oxygen equipment. The results from the expedition indicate that we were in error in three main areas.

First, we considerably underestimated the degree of hyperventilation (increased breathing). The effect this has on defending the level of oxygen in the lungs (Figure 7) is critical.

Next we underestimated the extent to which the pH of the blood would rise. This is partly determined by the hyperventilation, and partly by changes in blood chemistry brought about by the kidneys. The fact that the blood pH was much higher than we had predicted means that the lungs were better able to load oxygen, and this is also an appreciable advantage.

Finally, the barometric pressure was slightly higher than we had expected. Although the difference was not great, the amount of exercise a climber can do is so exquisitely sensitive to barometric pressure that this factor becomes significant.

An interesting and important question is to what extent is brain function affected by the marked derangement of the Po_2, Pco_2, and pH in the arterial blood. The degree of abnormality can be emphasized by pointing out that most patients with lung disease whose arterial Po_2 falls to 30 are likely to die.

Moreover, a P_{CO_2} as low as 7.5, and a pH higher than 7.7, are almost never seen in medical practice even in the most diseased patients. We are dealing here with conditions at the limit of human tolerance.

It is not surprising, therefore, that there are many examples of bad decisions being made at extreme altitudes, which indicate a befuddled state of mind. Occasional hallucinations have been described, such as that of F. S. Smythe in 1933. Other evidence of severe oxygen deprivation of the brain is the loss of peripheral vision. This is a bit like peering through a tunnel, and was described by Chris Chandler, M.D., when climbing high on Everest during the Bicentennial expedition of 1976.

It is little wonder that our psychometric tests showed clear evidence of brain impairment at Camp 2 and above, and, in the light of the summit findings, much less surprising that there was some residual brain damage detected after the expedition. Prospective climbers need to be aware of some of these possible consequences of going high, especially without supplementary oxygen.

9

SOLO!

"What life is for"[1]

Peter Hackett and Nuru Jangbo set off on their summit bid from Camp 5 about one hour after Chris Pizzo and Young Tenzing had left. This made their departure about 7:30 A.M. on October 24. However, they had not gone far before Nuru Jangbo's feet began to feel very cold, and he thought they were becoming frostbitten. He therefore returned to Camp 5. Reluctantly, Peter gave up all hope of getting to the summit, but because it was such a fine day he decided to walk slowly up the mountain some of the way, and meet Chris and Young Tenzing on their way down.

Peter takes up the story in this debriefing recorded when he returned to Camp 2.

HACKETT: I had no intention of going to the summit. I was having probably the most beautiful day of my life, you know, looking at all the mountains. I know almost all of them, but I never got to see them like that, and it was so warm. I was playing around with the radio trying to contact you guys at the time, but it wasn't warm enough. The radio didn't work too well.

See, when Nuru Jangbo left me I figured my summit chances were shot because I wouldn't have enough oxygen, and I'd have to solo because these guys weren't going to wait for me—they were way out ahead. I tried to catch up at one point, but couldn't, so I gave up, and the idea of soloing the Hillary Step was just ridiculous. So I said, fuck.[2] Why don't I just enjoy the most beautiful day of my life? I mean I was really into it.

So I was going kind of slow and leisurely and I just kept going. There was nothing better to do. The weather was so perfect you'd be a fool not to go as high as you could. So I figured I'd go to the South Summit and take some photographs, and rope up with these guys on the way back—because they could use another ice axe and it would just be safer. . . .

Well, I'm getting on to the South Summit, which was my goal for the day, when C-sahib [Pizzo] and Young Tenzing come down from the main summit and met me below the South Summit. I guess it was about 1:30, 1:40 in the afternoon.

PIZZO: It was actually 2, right at 2.

HACKETT: Was it right at 2 o'clock? And C-sahib gets on the radio, and starts talking to you [at Camp 2] about what a beautiful day it is and how Peter still has time to get up to the summit [murmurings in the background from Pizzo]—yeah, it's true! What, I do? Let's figure this out. I figured about another 40 minutes or so to the South Summit, or half an hour or so, and an hour and a half from the South Summit to the main summit and back.

PIZZO: I told him not to worry about the Hillary Step because the steps were in place.

HACKETT: Right. He said the steps were in place in the Hillary Step, and it wouldn't be too much trouble. You just have to be careful coming down. And then my little mind starts going, "holy shit, maybe I could actually climb Mt. Everest." Ha, ha, ha. And to help things,

128

Young Tenzing had two-thirds of a bottle of oxygen right there, and I had a quarter. Lack of oxygen was the other reason I figured I wouldn't go anywhere. So Young Tenzing and I switched oxygen bottles. I figured, "well, I'll go to the South Summit anyhow, take a look at it from there, you know."

Well, I don't know what it was but all of a sudden I woke up. I said, "Fuck, this is Mt. Everest. This isn't McKinley, or some shit you know. Why am I dillydallying all day long? Fuck. Just, I mean it must be high-altitude lassitude or my hippy mode. But look man, if you really pour it on you can do this fucker."

So I poured it on. I started moving a lot faster, and I got to the South Summit. I looked over there, and I could see the Hillary Step. It didn't look that bad. I could see the cornice ridge, a narrow ridge. It looked like you'd have to be very, very careful, and you'd have to really take your time and force yourself to think about your feet placement and your ice axe placement because you could easily end up in Tibet. So I said, what the hell, and I went for it. I didn't have a watch.

PIZZO: You didn't have a watch! I didn't know that. How could you know your turnaround time if you didn't have a watch? [Pizzo had made an arrangement with Hackett that the latter would turn around and descend no later than 4 P.M. irrespective of the altitude he had attained. Naturally, without a watch this arrangement did not mean much, hence Pizzo's astonishment.]

HACKETT: I was estimating! I broke my watch in the icefall. So, of course, I couldn't see the true summit from the South Summit. I thought I saw the true summit, but it went on longer, just like McKinley, or many peaks.

So I got to the Hillary Step pretty quickly, and it was terrible. The snow wouldn't hold a two-year-old. It wouldn't hold a baseball. It was just awful. But I noticed someone had cut out over to the left and had taken a more exposed route, but less steep and more solid, so I followed those tracks and got up in pretty good time. I was kind of scared because I wasn't belayed, and it wouldn't take much to . . . it was just slab snow and rock. I could have easily slipped right off.

So anyhow I got up in pretty good time and continued on, and there was . . . you had to be careful but it was actually nothing difficult . . . it actually felt good, because this was the first real climbing I had done on this expedition except for a little sherpa training and stuff. But I felt like I was a climber again, and that felt real nice. So, anyhow, I finally got to the summit, and stayed there about three minutes. I ran out of film, and it was real cold and windy, very, very windy.

While this was going on Chris Pizzo and Young Tenzing were descending from just below the South Summit, where they left Peter, to the old Camp 6 site. Chris had taken Peter's walkie talkie when Peter decided to head off alone, and before Chris and Young Tenzing set off on their descent to the old Camp 6 Chris called John Evans at Camp 2. The ensuing radio transmission was recorded, and tells the story. Remember that this is Chris's first contact with the rest of the expedition since he summited a couple of hours before.

PIZZO: Summit team to 2, do you read, over.

EVANS: Roger, summit team, we've got you loud and clear. Where are you? Over.

PIZZO: Please tell John West the barometric pressure on the summit of Everest is 253.0. Over.

EVANS: Copy, 253.0. [Cheers] Summit team, where are you now? Over.

PIZZO: Young Tenzing and I are descending. We are just below the South Summit where we met Peter Hackett who is ascending solo. Nuru Jangbo deserted him at 7:30 this morning with cold toes, and he's going to see how far he can get alone. He's only about an hour from the summit. I'm encouraging him to go ahead and go for it. Over.

EVANS: Well, I copy that, copy that. Are conditions safe enough, do you think? Over. [The transcript does not convey John's tone of voice, which is supportive but at the same time also concerned. He is obviously worried about Peter's safety.]

PIZZO: Conditions are very nice, probably just about what Kop encountered. Very little wind until you get to the South Summit, and then a moderate wind but not a big problem. The Hillary Step is beaten with good tracks now so I think there's no problem for a solo on the Hillary Step.

EVANS: Roger, got that. Are you going to wait there at the South Summit for him? Over.

PIZZO: We'll probably wait at the oxygen cache at Camp 6. Over.

EVANS: Okay, roger, I copied that. I understand. Is there some oxygen there at the cache? Over.

PIZZO: We saw a bunch of bottles. I haven't tried any yet. Over.

EVANS: Okay, C-sahib, that sounds good, sounds real good. We're a little bit . . . nervous having Peter up there so high by himself. Has he got oxygen left? Over.

PIZZO: He's got enough to get up. He'll run out on the way down. He's looking pretty good to me. I think he can go ahead. Over.

EVANS: Okay. I copied that. We'll be on pins and needles until we hear from all you guys later this afternoon. We'll keep monitoring our radio . . . just to hear what's going on. Over.

PIZZO: The rest of the data collection I think went very well. I collected six alveolar gas samples on the summit, and took a few pictures despite numb fingers. I'll hang around in the vicinity of Camp 6 waiting for Peter. Over.

EVANS: Okay, understand it. That's really good news, and
                we'll pass that on to Base. Anything else at this time?
                Over.

PIZZO: No, I'll get back to you when I sight Peter.

EVANS: Okay, as I say, we'll be listening. Peter, take care of
                yourself. Go very carefully, and we'll be monitoring
                the radio for news. Over.

PIZZO: Roger, summit team, over and out.

There is now a gap in the radio transmissions. John Evans had a chance
to mull over the implications of Peter going solo, and a short time later he
called up the summit team again.

EVANS: Camp 2 to summit team, do you copy?

PIZZO: I descended from the South Summit with Young Tenz-
                ing, and I am now waiting at the uppermost Camp 6,
                right on the ridge. A good vantage point for the South
                Summit and the main summit, although the summit
                route lies on the other side of the ridge so I can't
                really see Peter. I saw him disappear on the other
                side of the South Summit. I've been here about an
                hour. He said he would turn around at 4 o'clock at
                the latest. This would put him back at the South
                Summit at 5 o'clock, and get down here about 20
                minutes later. We have light, and can descend. I'm
                pretty confident we can descend—it is an easy slope
                to Camp 5—in 45 minutes or so. Over.

EVANS: C-sahib, we copied that. We'll stand by on the radio.
                Please let us know as soon as you see Peter coming.
                Over.

PIZZO: Roger, plan on doing that. Hopefully it will be within
                an hour or so. Over.

EVANS: Roger, sure hope so, we will be standing by. We're
                on pins and needles. So this is Camp 2 standing by.

PIZZO: Did you get some feedback yet from John West on
                    the barometer pressure at the summit? Is that about
                    what he expected or is that a little high? It seems high
                    to me. Over.

EVANS: We passed that to John West. What we got from him
                    was that he mostly was delighted that you got the
                    reading. I don't know if that was higher or lower than
                    he'd expected. Over.

PIZZO: Roger, Camp 2. I guess it can wait. I'll talk to him
                    about it later. Over until the sighting of Peter.

EVANS: Camp 2 standing by.

Meanwhile, Peter has been making his way down from the summit, and
he takes up the story shortly after his return to Camp 2.

HACKETT: I got some summit shots. Obviously there aren't any
                    pictures of me on the summit, which is a great loss.
                    So I started down and it was just steady, careful going.
                    I got to the Hillary Step, and I decided to go down
                    the other way instead of the way I came up, because
                    it looked like you could just sort of slip and slide your
                    way down. What a mistake. I mean there was a fair
                    amount of snow, you know. So you think you could
                    kick in deep enough, you think it would hold you.

                    So there I was, both feet dug in at about the same
                    level and my ice axe dug in in front of me, suddenly
                    realizing that none of the three points are solid, and
                    I fell. It was a huge shock. I thought, fuck it *was* that
                    kind of snow, just sugar. So I fell about maybe 10 or
                    15 feet, and landed with my lower leg locked in a
                    rocky crevasse. It was a good anchor, but I was upside
                    down, and the first thing I noticed was a massive
                    parasympathetic nervous system discharge—which
                    means that there was both feces and urine in my pants.
                    So I knew the situation was serious when that hap-
                    pened.

                    And then the next thing I noticed was that I was
                    hyperventilating tremendously. I was panicked. I ripped
                    off my oxygen mask because I felt claustrophobic,
                    and I don't know if that helped me at all. My goggles

133

went somewhere down in the Western Cwm. So there I was . . . and I still had my ice axe. I was hanging upside down with my knee caught.

So I tried to reach up with my ice axe and get something solid. Of course there wasn't anything solid. Finally I found a little wedge of rock that the pick of my ice axe stuck in, and with that I pulled myself upright. Just as I did that I saw a fixed line—from a previous expedition obviously . . . sort of back in the . . . what it is is a chimney, that's what it is, filled with snow. And what you really ought to do is just knock all the snow out of it, and then chimney on the rock or put in fixed lines. [Peter later pointed out that if he had not fallen, he would not have dislodged enough snow to uncover the fixed line.]

Anyhow, it was terrible rock, so I grabbed on to that line because I still didn't have a solid footing, just had a little of my ice axe in there. I finally got my knee out, and then I saw some steps not too far below me. Must have been Kop's steps in the snow.

I put my weight on that, but I fell through again. This time I fell about another 10 feet. But this time I ended up with one crampon on the rock, and I pushed off on it . . . you know, it was like a layback. I mean I was in the chimney actually, and I had my balance for a while anyhow. Then I saw the fixed line again back in there. So I grabbed onto the fixed line again and just held on to it, and let myself slide down another 10 or 15 feet. The snow was just fucking awful.

PIZZO: Was the fixed line to the left or right as you looked at the step?

HACKETT: Right. It was all old, you know. Finally, I got on to the steps, the solid steps at the bottom, that traverse, and got out. I was thinking they were C-sahib's. I didn't even trust those really. Because everything else had fallen apart on me. Gosh, it was terrible. Sugar, bottomless snow. Kop must have been able to pack it down enough at the time, but then a second person came along. No solidity whatsoever.

EVANS:

Kop . . . what he did was go up on the left. It was hard climbing with crampon points on the stratified rock and so forth. Coming down, he decided that well maybe with a belay he could kick good steps. He went down there making the steps as good as he could. However, Sungdare decided he didn't want any part of it, and Sungdare downclimbed the way they'd gone up.

HACKETT:

That's what I should have done. Those steps that he made . . . he was on belay. He probably just sort of slid down, you know. He didn't really make any decent steps. That would be my guess.

ANOTHER VOICE:

How difficult would it have been to come down the way you'd gone up?

HACKETT:

You know, it was good solid climbing and more stable. I could have done it. But it was more exposed, and I figured in this sort of chimney, I was, you know . . . more protected. I could just sort of slide down.

PIZZO:

It is more exposed, but there is less of an angle, and you can see better below when you're into the slope. You can stop each step and see where the next placement should be.

HACKETT:

Especially if you have an oxygen mask on. The chimney is so steep that you just can't see your next step down. So my mistake was I just started going down blind kicking. I think if I had to do it all over again I might just go down the Tibetan side—go over on that ridge.

PIZZO:

What! It's completely vertical.

HACKETT:

Yeah, but the snow is better. You know, it doesn't matter if it's absolutely vertical. I mean, if you can't see, just kick in and you know it's a good snow so you just go down. Anyhow, that exhausted me, thoroughly exhausted me, especially psychologically. You know, I figured it would get dark, I knew C-sahib wasn't going to come up here and look for me. If I'd hit my head on one of those pieces of rock that would have been it. It was not the most sane thing I've ever done. I mean, it wasn't even my idea. It was C-sahib's! I was just going to go to the South Summit and take some nice tourist pictures. . . .

PIZZO: He's exaggerating! I've got to tell you, the first thing he asked me was, can I give him an estimate on a round trip to the summit.

HACKETT: Well, I was naturally curious. Shit. I mean, here I was doing the South Summit, you know.

Meanwhile, below the South Summit Chris is waiting for Peter. Chris had a three-and-a-half-hour wait—from about 2:30 till 6 P.M. But he made good use of the time.

First of all, he collected another series of alveolar gas samples—these gave the data point labeled 8,400 meters in Figure 6. Although these samples were taken some 400 meters (1,300 feet) below the summit samples, in some respects they turned out to be more valuable. The samples taken at the summit showed abnormally high values for the "respiratory exchange ratio," a technical derivation based on the measured Po_2 and Pco_2 of the alveolar gas. This indicated that Pizzo was not in a steady state of gas exchange when the samples were taken. We are not sure of the reason for this; it may simply be that he had so much to do during his 30 minutes on the summit that he could not settle down into a resting state. Another possibility is that there was lactic acid in his blood following the exertions of the climb to the summit. In any case, this high respiratory exchange ratio means that the interpretation of the summit values is uncertain.

By contrast, the measurements taken at the old Camp 6 were excellent from a technical point of view. The value for respiratory exchange ratio was normal, which may reflect the fact that Chris had all the time in the world to take the samples. Chris also carried out measurements of resting ventilation using the flow meter, but unfortunately the Medilog recorder had stopped by this time, and no useful data were obtained.

Chris was well aware of the dangers involved in waiting so long for Peter, as the tape that he recorded at the time shows.

"Time is 3 o'clock. I've descended to the uppermost Camp 6 at about the same elevation of Lhotse, whatever that may be. I've sent what's-his-name Tenzing on down, and I'm waiting here for Peter who is making a brave and

136

foolhardy summit bid. While I'm waiting here for Peter I've decided to take six alveolar gas samples and record another pressure and temperature which was . . . just a minute please . . . barometric pressure was 267.1, temperature minus 9.4. I figure I'm only 300 feet or so above my first pressure/temperature check of this morning.

"Now I've been here for about half an hour. It's 3:06 right now, let's say I was here at 2:30 so we'll notice a drop in heart rate then. At 2 o'clock I met up with Peter, and he gave me a Dexedrine, so if you notice any cardiographic irregularities from here on out you may want to take that into account. Just to synchronize the Medilog, I'm going to push event marker number 3 right now. It is 3:07:40.

"Now I thought it might be interesting . . . it's 3:08:10 . . . I just signed back on again to do spirometry while at rest. I've been off O s [oxygen] for about five minutes, still feel kind of breathless. Let's do spirometry for five minutes, green for go and red for stop. This is spirometry at rest, whether you're interested or not.

"Okay it's 3:16. I just completed spirometry as planned. I feel I was adequately oxygenated at rest. Now I'm not lightheaded at all. There was a little increased inspiratory resistance compared to what I recall. I believe only two or three leaflets on the intake valve were functional, but it didn't cramp my style at rest at all.

"Now I'll continue to wait for Peter. I'm out of food and out of water, but I'm well clothed and feel I can make Camp 5 in an hour, but I'm not leaving here until dark. If I don't make it down and someone discovers this tape . . . it's very important . . . please return it to Dr. John West, Department of Physiology, School of Medicine, University of California, San Diego, La Jolla, California."

At about 5 o'clock in the afternoon John Evans called Chris Pizzo again on the radio.

EVANS: Camp 2 to summit party, do you copy?

PIZZO: You're all static. Will you try that again, over.

EVANS: Receiving you loud and clear. Go ahead.

PIZZO: Okay, got you that time John. I just sighted Peter at the South Summit. The hard part of the climb is over for him. He should be joining me in about half an hour. Then another hour after that to Camp 5. Chances are 90 percent he made the summit. I'll confirm that when he gets here. Over.

EVANS: Roger, we've been very anxious, very anxious for Peter. We're glad that you've got a visual on him, and will continue to monitor the radio. How are you doing? Are you staying warm? Over.

PIZZO: Starting to cool down . . . fingers and toes. I can hang on long enough until he gets here. I've got plenty of clothes. The wind seems nice in this particular spot, and also there's the sun. I don't think there's any problem. He'll be here in half an hour. Over.

EVANS: Roger, that sounds great. That's terrific news. Again congratulations to you both. Another question. Is there oxygen there? Over.

PIZZO: I just checked the Luxfer tanks at the upper Camp 6. They are all empty. I did leave a bottle as planned on the way up at this spot, and it's half full, so I'm fine. I think Peter is fine too, because as Young Tenzing and I were coming down we met him going up. He was down to about a quarter of a tank. He traded with Young Tenzing who had about two-thirds of a tank. So I think we're fine back to 5. Over.

EVANS: Okay, roger. That's terrific news. As I've said we've been quite anxious for both of you, and we'll continue to stand by the radio until you and Peter lock up. Again, we're all delighted because we've been here wringing our hands for the last couple of hours. So we'll stand by. Stay warm in the meantime.

Several of us at Base Camp were monitoring the radio transmissions when we could. At this point I called John Evans.

WEST: Base Camp to Camp 2, do you copy, John?

EVANS: Roger, Base Camp, you're loud and clear.

WEST: I just came in at the end of that transmission, and couldn't hear what it was. Could you just summarize it for us please?

EVANS:	Roger. We had C-sahib loud and clear. He had just observed Peter Hackett coming to the South Summit on the way down. C-sahib is waiting below at the Bicentennial Camp 6. Says he's beginning to get a bit cold, but he's going to wait there. He thinks Peter will join him there in about half an hour. In another hour from there they'll be safely back at 5. He thinks that there's a very good chance that Peter Hackett reached the summit, but that is just conjecture at this time. Do you copy?
WEST:	Yes, copied that John. That's tremendous news that Peter showed up . . . that's just marvelous news . . . okay. The summit I don't mind so much, but the fact that he's safe is just so marvelous. Let's see. Why don't we have another sked one hour from now, which would be 6 o'clock.
EVANS:	Right, I copy, John, and I concur with your thoughts, and we'll expect your call at 6 o'clock. By that time we should know whether Peter summited, and also we should get a confirmation that they are in fact okay.

There is another gap in radio transmissions until 6 o'clock. At that time Pizzo calls Camp 2.

PIZZO:	Summit team to Camp 2, come in. Over.
EVANS:	Yes, we have you loud and clear. Go ahead.
PIZZO:	Peter has just arrived at Camp 6. He did make the summit. Quite an epic. He survived a fall at the Hillary Step. He's pretty wasted. I'll put him on my rope, and get him down in what remaining light there is. We'll give you a call shortly after our arrival at Camp 5.
EVANS:	Did Peter make the summit?
PIZZO:	Affirmative. Peter made the summit. Peter made a grand solo today. We have two sets of Medilog data. Over.

139

EVANS: [Cheers] Hey listen, we're really proud of you guys. There are a lot of details we'd like to know, but we'll get them later, tomorrow or whenever. Go back and get yourselves warm, and give us a call later this evening if you feel like it.

At 8 P.M. John Evans called Chris Pizzo again.

EVANS: Hello, Camp 5, this is 2. Do you copy?

PIZZO: Yeah. Do you read me?

EVANS: Roger, do. How are you guys doing up there by now?

PIZZO: Just pulled in—an epic descent in the pitch black. Wish Karl could have ordered us up a moon. But we made it back, and we're getting ready to hydrate back up and to go to bed.

EVANS: Great, terrific. Are your fingers and toes and everything okay?

PIZZO: All three of us are healthy. Peter and I are just quite exhausted and dehydrated. Especially Peter. Peter deserves a hell of a lot of credit for a solo ascent of a more difficult than expected route.

MARET: Roger, we copy you. We're all cheering down below at Base Camp and up here for that incredible feat that you did, especially Peter. Can you tell me what are your plans in the morning?

PIZZO: Yeah, we're going to sleep in.

EVANS: Roger, that sounds good.

PIZZO: We can do a couple of items of South Col science. If it's not windy in the morning we can set up the bicycle. If it is windy we'll probably stick each other for blood specimens, and come down. Over.

140

EVANS: Roger, copy that. That sounds real good, C-sahib, real good. We'll be anxious to see you when you get down, and we'll be monitoring the radio every hour. When you wake up, and when the spirit moves you, give us a call. Over.

PIZZO: Will do, John, probably between 8 and 9 when the sun hits the tent. Over.

EVANS: Okay, roger. Again, congratulations on a marvelous achievement, and have a good night.

PIZZO: Okay, thank you for your congratulations, and congratulations to you, John, and to John West, and all the guys down below who busted their butts putting in this difficult route, and the camps on the headwall. This is for all you guys. Over.

EVANS: Okay, roger. Thanks for that . . . very gracious comments. Camp 2 out.

At this point Chris recorded the last section of the dictation tape that he took to the summit.

                          "The time is 8:09. Dr. Peter and myself just got back to the tent. I am now going to turn off the Med-ilog, and start putting fluids and all kinds of exotic things in my body to make it feel better. I was happy to have this opportunity to do this work for you, Dr. West. You better make something out of it!"

The descent from the old Camp 6 to Camp 5 took 2 hours. Chris and Peter started in fading light, but after 10 minutes they were in pitch darkness just as though they had been covered by a big black blanket, as Chris put it. There was no moon. Fortunately Peter had a headlamp, and he led with Chris coming along behind a full length of rope away.

Peter described it thus:

141

HACKETT: We had that epic descent to the South Col. Actually, we were in pretty good shape. We knew basically how to find Camp 5. It was very windy, but we were both dressed well, and it wasn't all that cold. We were lucky. I mean, that's the whole reason I went for it, because conditions were so good . . . I was so exhausted that I'd start glissading. I'd just sit down and let myself go. I mean, after a while I couldn't even hang onto that because the snow was too hard. Didn't have enough strength to get down. I was really blown. I mean, if I had planned on a summit attempt I'd have psyched myself up more, had a little more water and gone faster instead of just strolling to the South Summit. And now that's all over. You know I'm left with . . .

EVANS: Fame, glory, and money.

HACKETT: Money? Not even fame and glory.

The following morning Chris and Peter did additional scientific measurements. First they each took another series of alveolar gas samples. The results were fascinating—they showed that both climbers were now breathing less than the subjects who had contributed the alveolar gas samples at Camp 5 on October 12, one day after Camp 5 had been established. The data from Chris are particularly interesting because he was a subject on both occasions. His P_{CO_2} had a mean value of 9.0 on October 12, but 12.5 at the same altitude on the morning after his successful summit climb thirteen days later.

The reasons for this increase are not fully understood. One suggestion was that the tremendous amount of breathing that both climbers did during their summit climb may have resulted in some fatigue of the respiratory muscles. This phenomenon of an increase in P_{CO_2} because of respiratory fatigue has been noted in marathon runners after a hard race.

Even more important than the alveolar gas samples were samples of venous blood taken at the same time. Special syringes had been prepared by Bob Winslow, but even so it was no small feat to remove blood from each other's arm veins under the trying conditions of Camp 5. The samples were immediately placed in an ice-water slurry inside a vacuum (Dewar) flask, and given to sherpas who took them rapidly down the fixed rope to Camp 2.

When they arrived there several hours later Bob Winslow carried out various analyses. These included a measurement of "base excess," a number that indicates how effectively the kidney has responded to the increased alkalinity of the blood as a result of the hyperventilation. It was astonishing how little the kidneys had compensated, and the net result was a very high pH (extreme alkalinity) in the arterial blood on the summit, as discussed in the last chapter. This suggestive evidence that this aspect of kidney function is dramatically impaired at these extreme altitudes should be followed up.

Finally, what can be said of Peter's solo ascent? Very few climbers have reached the summit of Everest solo, and fewer still have returned to tell the tale. The most remarkable was Reinhold Messner's solo ascent from the north without supplementary oxygen in 1980. That feat stands in a class by itself. It is probable that Mick Burke reached the summit during Bonington's successful southwest face expedition of 1975, but he was never seen again. It is presumed that he slipped and fell on his way down in a blizzard that began suddenly and enveloped the mountain. In addition, Franz Oppurg made a successful solo summit climb from the South Col during the 1978 Austrian expedition. Thus Peter's was the third documented solo ascent.

Peter's decision to make a solo attempt on the summit at 2 o'clock in the afternoon when he was still some distance below the South Summit could well be called "foolhardy," to use Chris Pizzo's word. Yet, knowing Peter, it was not completely surprising. Peter is something of a loner, and I never got to know him well. I once asked him why he chose to spend so much time at the Himalayan Rescue Association Clinic in Pheriche, a remote village a few days' walk below the Everest Base Camp. He half jokingly replied that he came from a family of ten brothers, and reveled in the opportunity to get away from everybody. Certainly at Pheriche he spent many months in the company of only a few sherpas. There is another side to Peter that I never clearly saw. He once spent some time in a Jesuit seminary, and I sensed a thoughtful, contemplative attitude that Peter kept rather private. There is an earnestness too about his manner that suggests hidden qualities.

There have been several discussions since the expedition about who was responsible for Peter's decision to go solo. Of course, ultimately he was, but the elation of Chris having just come down from the summit must have been a factor. Naturally, since everything turned out well, there were no recriminations. Why not let Mallory have the last word: "If you cannot understand that there is something in man which responds to the challenge of this mountain and goes to meet it, that the struggle is the struggle of life itself upward and forever upward, then you won't see why we go. . . . What we get from this adventure is just sheer joy. . . . That is what life means and what life is for."

10

RETURN

"A more grosse and temperate aire"[1]

Chris Pizzo and Peter Hackett returned to Camp 2 on the afternoon of October 25, and walked down to Base Camp on the 27th. The rest of the expedition who had been up at Camp 2 gradually filtered in, and we had a celebration meal of delicacies that had been donated to the expedition and had unaccountably survived for two months in the storehouse. These included smoked oysters, several jars of caviar, and some beer.

The fact that such gourmet items could still be found at Base Camp underlined the rather curious selection of food that we had on the expedition. As indicated earlier, most of the food had been donated—not the best way of ensuring a balanced diet. For example, we were very short of canned beef which is an acceptable staple food for long periods in remote areas, as many a G.I. will attest. On the other hand, we were not the first expedition to include delicacies in our rations. When Ang Pema's fare hit rock bottom, I occasionally got vicarious pleasure by recalling that the supplies on the 1924 Everest expedition included sixty cans of quail in foie gras and four dozen bottles of champagne!

John Evans has a great love of mountains, and he was adamant that we leave the route cleaner than we found it; he supervised a big cleanup operation.

145

Virtually all evidence of the camps and climbing equipment was removed or burned; there was a spectacular bonfire up at Camp 2. The only remaining items were the damaged tents at Camp 5, and some fixed rope on the headwall between Camp 5 and the Cwm. Everything else, including all the ropes and ladders in the icefall, was taken out. Prior to the expedition someone had proposed a study of our environmental impact on the Everest area. John assured him that this would be a waste of time in our case, and he was correct.

Some mail arrived on the 27th. I was hoping for news of my wife, Penny. We had arranged that she would try to walk in to Base Camp at the end of the expedition, but so far I had heard little. There were two strange telegrams. One was from Richard Blum of San Francisco asking me to send him news of the American Expedition on the east face of Everest. We didn't have any information about what was happening on the other side of the mountain; that expedition could have been on the far side of the moon for all we knew. The other telegram was from the Perlman family wishing us luck and happy birthday to their son, Eric, a member of the east face expedition.

I suppose the reason these telegrams were sent to us was the hope that we had radio contact with the east face group. There was no way that our VHF radios could get around Mt. Everest; the frequencies that we were using (151 MHz) were good only for near line-of-sight contacts. Incidentally, I realized during the expedition that the common practice of taking handy talkie 2 meter radios for links between camps is not ideal. Since the vast majority of the messages have to be transmitted between fixed sites, it would be much better to use high-gain directional antennas rather than the little stubs that stick out of the top of the handheld transceivers.

While the mountain was being cleared of equipment, the Base Camp laboratory was a hive of activity with Frank Sarnquist, Brownie Schoene, and Peter Hackett completing the hemodilution study. This was briefly described at the end of Chapter 6, the objective being to determine whether reducing the red-cell concentration in the blood to more nearly normal levels improved exercise capacity or brain function.

We had a scare when the study was carried out on Dave Graber, the last of the four subjects. He developed a reaction to the injected albumin solution with a skin rash and mild fever. Such a reaction is extremely rare, but it brought home to us that an invasive procedure in such a remote environment can easily turn into a serious unpleasant situation because there was little if any way to treat him. Fortunately the reaction was short-lived. But then, perhaps to remind us how lucky we had been during the last three months, fate dealt us another surprise. Big D developed an infection in his arm at the site of the injection. This too was unexpected, because we were using presterilized equip-

146

ment. It was ironic that this was virtually the last venipuncture of perhaps 100 that had been carried out during the scientific program, and the only one to give rise to complications.

Bob Winslow decided that it would be valuable to have some additional data on the composition of sherpa blood. As indicated in Chapter 6, this has been a confusing area because some previous measurements suggested that the sherpas are different from high-altitude natives of other areas of the world. Bob explained to sirdar Sonam Girme that he needed some volunteers, whereupon Sonam blew his whistle and the sherpas dutifully lined up outside the laboratory. However, when they saw the syringes and needles being prepared for the venipunctures, there was some shuffling of feet, and many of them disappeared. Nevertheless, Bob was able to get samples from thirteen of them. These measurements were very valuable; they showed that sherpa blood physiology is essentially no different from that of Andean high-altitude dwellers.

The highlight of October 28 for me was a note from Penny to say that she and several other wives and friends of the expedition were heading for Lobuya, and hoped to reach Base Camp the following day. On the basis of this I had a shower, the first for over a month. Ang Pema warmed the water in the kitchen, but the air temperature on the glacier was extremely cold and the whole experience was frigid. Brownie, who was also expecting his wife, Marsha, also had a shower but subsequently announced rather ungallantly that no woman was worth that! Needless to say the remark was not to be taken seriously.

People often ask about the washing arrangements on the expedition. The answer is that at Base Camp it was possible to have an occasional shower, and in fact we had brought in a special kit for this purpose. It consisted of a bag of black plastic with a tube and a pinch clip attached, and the idea was to heat the water by exposing it to the midday sun. We also had a more elaborate solar water heater. However, the surest way to get enough hot water was to ask Ang Pema to heat some.

At Camp 2 it was impossible to wash except for hands and face. In fact, it was essentially impossible to undress because of the cold, and you were fated to wear the same underclothes for several weeks from leaving Base Camp until returning. The best plan then was to burn them.

After lunch the next day Sonam announced that the wives and friends were on their way up the Khumbu Glacier from Gorak Shep. It was always a mystery to me how the sherpas seemed to know precisely what was happening several miles away in spite of not receiving any direct news as far as I could tell. Nevertheless, I set off down the Glacier to meet Penny, and it was a wonderful experience to see her looking so well in spite of her unexpectedly rapid ascent from Lukla.

147

Prior to the expedition Penny had arranged a trek of wives and friends to meet the expedition as we walked out. She put together a party of six people including Marsha Schoene, Nancy Winslow, Miranda (now married to Chris Pizzo), Karen, a friend of Karl's, and Jim Swanson, an old friend of the Schoenes.

The party flew to Lukla at an altitude of about 2,800 meters (9,200 feet), and gradually made their way to Namche and then up the Dudh Kosi and Imja Khola valleys through Thyangboche and Pheriche on their way to Base Camp. The sherpa in charge of the trek was Lakpar, along with Ang Kami, their cook. The two sherpas arranged for several porters to carry the loads so that the group had only small day packs.

The party spent Thursday night at Base Camp, but the following morning Brownie Schoene, Bob Winslow, and myself, with Marsha, Nancy, and Penny walked down to Gorak Shep. Brownie and I scrambled up Kala Pattar to take the classical photograph of the southwest face of Everest in perfect light. It was the same view that Charlie Houston and his group had seen way back in 1950 when the first westerners coming through Nepal had spotted the potential route to Everest from the south, and I pondered briefly on the dramatic events that had occurred here in the last thirty years. The view has been the subject of innumerable photographs since then by Everest aficionados who often make this the culmination of their trek.

That evening Brownie, Bob, and I began to realize how pleasant a Mountain Travel trek was compared with an expedition. The delicious meal was served with all the trimmings, including a tablecloth, a lamp, and a bowl of hand-washing water outside the tent. It was cold that night, but as Penny and I lay in our sleeping bags listening to the Schubert Trout Quintet on Penny's Walkman, life seemed very good indeed.

We were called at 6 A.M., which seemed unnecessarily spartan, but apparently that is the tradition on Mountain Travel treks. That day we walked slowly down to Pheriche, stopping for a delicious omelet lunch at Lobuya. It was marvelous to walk down into the thicker air knowing that most of the problems of the expedition were behind. After two months of nothing but ice and rock, the sight and smell of green plants was delicious. I can vividly remember the first mosslike growth that we saw as we emerged from the moraine just before Gorak Shep.

The rest of the expedition arrived at Pheriche on November 1. Peter Hackett had arranged a mammoth party in the Himalayan Rescue Association Clinic. Peter had somehow found a large number of bottles of Nepalese Star beer, and drinking and dancing started during the afternoon. After it got dark there was traditional sherpa dancing outside. The sherpas formed a large circle with interlocking arms, and slowly moved their feet in an intricate rhythm that is surprisingly difficult to follow either before or after you have been drinking chang, a fermented beerlike beverage. There was an enormous cask of chang in the center of the group, and several old sherpanis handed around cups of it, encouraging us to drink.

The following day we walked on to Thyangboche, now a hive of activity in contrast to the peace and quiet when we arrived two months before. Brightly colored tents were everywhere, and there was even a restaurant. John Evans and Sonam Girme arrived, and we had another audience with the chief lama. Sonam told him how successful the expedition had been, and we thanked him for his spiritual support. How right he had been—we had certainly had more than our share of luck.

En route to Thyangboche, Penny and I passed the spot where the leader of a Swiss expedition to Lhotse Shar fell to his death some weeks before. It was a strange story. First there had been tragedy on the mountain when two of the expedition members had died after turning back less than 250 meters (800 feet) from the summit. Then on the way out, the leader, Joseph Fauchere, had been walking along this narrow but heavily traveled trail when he fell down the steep slope into the valley below. We never did determine the cause of the accident

In the evening Penny and I walked out along the ridge near the monastery to see the memorial to Jack Breitenbach, the young climber killed in the ice-fall during the 1963 American Everest expedition. The memorial has a spectacular setting—the deep ravine of the Imja Khola in the center, Ama Dablam magnificent on the right, and the Everest massif on the left. This has to be one of the greatest views in the world.

Next day we walked down to Namche Bazar. En route Penny and I decided to have lunch at the Hotel Everest View. This hotel, built by an enterprising Japanese businessman, has a magnificent view of Everest, Taweche, and Ama Dablam, and it has its own private airport at Thyangboche. It was a steep pull up to the hotel. When we arrived we were taken aback to find that they were not serving lunch. The reason was that there were no guests—one of their aircraft had crashed a few days before and no guests could be flown in. However, they generously put together a meal for the Winslows and ourselves. It was very elegant with a linen tablecloth, china, and silver. We were also able to read a *Herald Tribune* of a few days previously, and I was interested to see that nothing much seemed to have happened while we were away. We were shown one of the hotel rooms. It was attractive, with a big picture window view. I had heard that oxygen is piped into the rooms because the altitude of the hotel is very high at about 3,800 meters (12,500 feet), and it is possible to

149

fly directly in from Kathmandu. However this is not the case, though tanks of oxygen can be rolled into the room if required. This is certainly better than the arrangement on the Peruvian trains going over the Andes where, I am told, the conductor will blow oxygen at your face from a rubber bag for a small consideration.

The next evening there was a big farewell party at Sonam Girme's beautiful house in Namche Bazar. It was surprisingly formal, with all the expedition members sitting around a long table. The food was yak steak and enormous quantities of delicious rakshi and chang. A large number of kartas (white scarves) were given out; this is a traditional ceremony during a celebration. The meal was followed by prodigious drinking. There was a group of toothless old sherpanis whose job was to take around jugs of chang and apply considerable social pressure to have each member finish one at a gulp. We all got back to our beds safely, and there were surprisingly few hangovers in the morning. I did see Brownie hobbling around, but he emphasized that he had sprained his ankle *before* the party.

The following day Penny and I walked down to Lukla to see if we could get a flight home. We found chaos—over 300 people were waiting, including Larry Lahiri, who had been sitting around for the last four days. He was annoyed because he had a solid reservation several days ago. This airstrip is frequently closed by low clouds that roll in from the valley. On this occasion there had been almost no flights for several days, and tempers were starting to fray.

Fortunately the Royal Nepalese Airline Corporation declared a state of emergency, and diverted a number of their Twin Otter STOL aircraft to Lukla to clear the backlog. As luck would have it, Penny managed to get a flight at a few minutes' notice the following day, and she went out clutching the valuable box of expedition data and alveolar gas samples. I was able to follow the next day after spending a very comfortable night at the Sherpa Cooperative Hotel where the room cost me $10, which I thought exorbitant at the time. Some of the expedition members showed up there for an evening meal, and it was a pleasure to watch them eat. Several ordered two servings of the main course and still felt hungry. We all had enormous appetites as we got down to this oxygen-rich environment of only 2,800 meters (9,200 feet).

I got out of Lukla the next day, and joined Penny at the Hotel Malla in Kathmandu. Here we had a busy five days. Dr. Brenda Townes had flown in from Seattle to carry out the postexpedition psychometric measurements and, as explained in Chapter 6, she found several residual abnormalities. I spent some time with John Evans going over the events of the expedition, and checking with him on the dates of establishing the camps and the various altitudes. I was astonished that there were already some differences of opinion on the details of what happened, and I was glad that I had kept a copious diary, and that I had the tapes of the debriefing sessions of the three summiters.

One amusing example of differences of opinion occurred later, after we had returned to the U.S., when I sent out a note to members giving them our best estimates of the heights of the camps. These were chiefly based on the barometric pressure measurements. The table is included in Appendix B. I got back two dissenting opinions by return mail, both disputing the altitude of Camp 5. One of the summiters said it was certainly lower; the other climber (who did not go above 5) was equally certain it was higher!

In fact, we can be confident that the altitude was very close to 8,050 meters (26,400 feet). We have barometric pressure measurements on six separate days giving this altitude. In addition, two summiters estimated it to be about "200 feet" (61 meters) above the South Col, the altitude of which is accurately known as 7,986 meters (26,200 feet).

Incidentally, our altitude for Camp 2, namely 6,300 meters (20,700 feet), is considerably below some estimates by previous expeditions. Again our figure is based on 35 measurements of barometric pressure and is certainly very close. It seems that previous expeditions have often overestimated the altitude of this camp,

John and I spent a couple of interesting hours talking to Elizabeth Hawley who was a mine of information not only about current events in the Himalaya but also about previous expeditions. She told us that there were 40 expeditions in Nepal in that postmonsoon season. These resulted in 12 deaths, and at least 6 of these could be attributed to the storm at the end of September that had kept us immobilized for several days. I also had various interviews with the press.

Our remaining logistic problem was getting the frozen blood samples that had been inadvertently left at the Camp 2 laboratory back to the United States. The main group of samples had been taken back in special containers by Duane Blume. We had our samples stored in a freezer in the American compound in Kathmandu, but could not find dry ice in which to pack the shipment. Telex messages to Calcutta had not been answered. It was also essential to find somebody who was going straight back to California so that the samples would not thaw out en route. I delegated this problem to Rick Peters who had not yet arrived in Kathmandu; he dealt with it with his usual efficiency, and brought the samples back intact. He told us later that all the large aircraft have dry ice on board for keeping food cold, so this did not turn out to be a problem after all.

On November 11 John and I had our formal postexpedition meeting with the Ministry of Tourism. And that afternoon I gave the first of what turned out to be a series of lectures about our expedition. The audience was a group of doctors at the Bir Hospital in Kathmandu, the main teaching hospital. Although they could hardly be expected to have a particular interest in the physiology of extreme altitudes (as a medical problem in a developing country like Nepal this must be an extremely low priority!) the response was lively.

That evening the American ambassador to Nepal, Carl Kool, gave a splendid party for the expedition. The extensive guest list included many government officials, including the Honorable Drona S. J. B. Rana, Minister of State for Tourism, and Inspector Yogendra Thapa, our first liaison officer who succeeded in reaching Camp 5, much to his credit. There were also physicians from Bir Hospital and Shanta Bhawan Hospital. (The latter is a Christian mission hospital in Kathmandu. The staff gave us a great deal of support during the 1960–61 expedition.) A large group from the American embassy included Robert Goold, who had helped us with our customs problems when we first arrived in Kathmandu, and a galaxy of diplomats from other embassies including France, Great Britain, Federal Republic of Germany, and the People's Republic of China. It was a fine night.

On the following day John Evans, Penny, and I started our long flight back to the United States. After a night in Bangkok we arrived in Seattle, having had two Friday the 13ths. It was a marvelous day for me—I saw my children Joanna and Robert for the first time in almost four months. There was a tremendous welcome at San Diego airport, with the UCSD laboratory turning out in force.

As I write this more than a year later, the elation of this great adventure still remains. Of course we were an extremely lucky expedition. The fact that Chris Pizzo found an ice axe at just the right time so that he could get to the summit and make his scientific measurements is stranger than fiction. And Peter Hackett's miraculous escape after his accident on the Hillary Step is still hard to believe.

The scientific data from the expedition exceeded all our expectations. In retrospect, we see that some additional measurements could have been done, but we did not realize their importance at the time. Nevertheless, the total of the successful measurements was far more than we had any right to expect. Appendix C contains a preliminary list of scientific articles from the expedition. Is it ungracious for me to hope that it will be seen by the three members of the Study Section who voted to disapprove that critical grant back in 1979!

There were several articles about the expedition in various newspapers and magazines with various degrees of accuracy. The most surprising was an informative article in the Russian newspaper, *Soviet Sport*, of March 31, 1982.

Apparently this has a vast circulation, and it was odd to find the expedition more widely reported in the Soviet Union than the U.S.

In the fall of 1982, just a year after the expedition ended, we had a reunion in the Rocky Mountains outside Denver. Brownie put together a great program with some scientific presentations; there was a clever spoof on the science by Mike Weis, and a good deal of reminiscing. Just prior to that we had a symposium on "High Altitude and Man" at the fall meeting of the American Physiological Society in San Diego. Much of the material for the symposium came from our expedition, and this was published in a book of the same name in the Clinical Physiology series of the American Physiological Society.

For me personally the expedition was the experience of a lifetime. Although my work is stimulating enough, and our laboratory is very productive, the weight of administrative and other humdrum responsibilities is enough to make anyone wonder whether this is what life is really about. As therapy for a midlife crisis, the opportunity to help to put together a medical research expedition to the highest mountain in the world is hard to beat. Certainly things will never be the same.

NOTES

Chapter 1

1. The remark was apparently made by George Mallory in 1923 in response to an American reporter who asked him why he wanted to climb Mt. Everest.

2. A little poetic license has been taken with the order of Pizzo's activities here on the summit. For a full, accurate account see Chapter 8.

3. This fine quotation was included in Thomas F. Hornbein, *Everest: The West Ridge* (San Francisco: Sierra Club, 1963). I have not been able to find the original source.

Chapter 2

1. From I. Acosta, *The Naturall and Morall Historie of the East and West Indies* (London, Edward Blount and William Aspley, 1604), p. 148. (The relevant section is reprinted in J. B. West, ed., *High Altitude Physiology* [Stroudsburg, Pa.: Hutchinson, Ross Publishing Company, 1981], which contains many historical papers on high-altitude physiology, as well as extracts of all the papers cited in notes 1 through 10 of this chapter.)

2. Ibid.

3. See A. Wylie, "Notes on the Western Regions," *Journal of the Royal Anthropological Institute* 10 (1881): 36–38.

4. See J. Glaisher, ed., *Travels in the Air* (Philadelphia: J.B. Lippincott, 1871), pp. 50–58.

5. See P. Bert, *Barometric Pressure: Researches in Experimental Physiology*, trans. M. A. and F. A. Hitchcock (Columbus, Ohio: College Book Company, 1943).

6. The "partial pressure" of a gas is obtained by multiplying the total pressure by the concentration of the gas. For example, dry air at sea level (barometric pressure 760 mm mercury) has an oxygen concentration of 21 percent, and therefore a partial

pressure (Po_2) of 160 mm mercury. When dry air is inhaled into the lung airways, water vapor is added with a partial pressure of 47 mm mercury, and the partial pressure of the dry air is reduced by this amount. A climber on the summit of Mt. Everest, where the barometric pressure is 253 mm mercury, will have a true inspired Po_2 of $(253 - 47) \times 21/100 = 43$ mm mercury.

7. See C. G. Douglas et al., "Physiological Observations Made on Pike's Peak, Colorado, with Special Reference to Adaptations to Low Barometric Pressures," *Phil. Trans. Royal Soc.*, ser. B, 203 (1913): 185–381.

8. See J. Barcroft, "Observations upon the Effect of High Altitude on the Physiological Processes of the Human Body, Carried out in the Peruvian Andes, Chiefly at Cerro de Pasco," *Phil. Trans. Royal Soc.*, ser. B, 211 (1923): 351–480.

9. See C. Monge, *Acclimatization in the Andes* (Baltimore: Johns Hopkins Press, 1948).

10. See A. Keyes, "The Physiology of Life at High Altitudes: The International High Altitude Expedition to Chile, 1953," *Scientific Monthly* 43 (1936): 289–312.

11. The expedition is described in Edmund Hillary and Desmond Doig, *High in the Thin, Cold Air* (New York: Doubleday, 1962), and in *National Geographic*, October 1962, pp. 503–47. The scientific program was described by L. G. C. E. Pugh in *British Medical Journal* 2 (1962): 621–27.

12. See C. S. Houston, "Operation Everest: A Study of Acclimatization to Anoxia," *U.S. Naval Med. Bull.* 46 (1946): 1783–92.

13. See J. B. West and P. D. Wagner, "Predicted Gas Exchange on the Summit of Mount Everest," *Resp. Physiol.* 42 (1980): 1–16.

Chapter 3

1. Quoted in H. W. Tilman, *Mount Everest 1938* (Cambridge: University Press, 1948), p. 125.

Chapter 4

1. From C. K. Howard-Bury, *Mount Everest: The Reconnaissance, 1921* (London: Edward Arnold, 1922), p. 184.

2. Ibid.

Chapter 5

1. From E. Hillary, *High Adventure* (London: Hodder and Stoughton, 1955), p. 50. The subsequent quotation is also from this source.

Chapter 6

1. From I. Acosta, *The Naturall and Morall Historie of the East and West Indies* (London: Edward Blount and William Aspley, 1604), p. 148.

2. For more information about some of the scientific equipment used on the expedition, see K. Maret, "Expedition to Mount Everest, 1981: Technical Aspects," in J. R.

Sutton et al., eds., *Hypoxia: Man at Altitude* (New York: Thieme-Stratton, 1982), pp. 125–29.

3. For a summary of the research program, see J. B. West, "Human Physiology at Extreme Altitudes on Mount Everest," *Science* 223 (February 24, 1984): 784–88.

4. See J. B. West and P. D. Wagner, "Predicted Gas Exchange on the Summit of Mount Everest," *Resp. Physiol.* 42 (1980): 1–16.

5. For a full account, see J. B. West et al., "Maximal Exercise at Extreme Altitudes on Mount Everest," *J. Appl. Physiol.: Respirat. Environ. Exercise Physiol.* 55 (1983): 688–98.

6. See S. Lahiri et al., "Dependence of High Altitude Sleep Apnea on Ventilatory Sensitivity to Hypoxia," *Resp. Physiol.* 52 (1983): 281–301.

7. See R. M. Winslow et al., "Red Cell Function at Extreme Altitude on Mount Everest," *J. Appl. Physiol.: Resp. Environ. Exercise Physiol.* 56 (1984): 109–16.

8. F. H. Sarnquist et al., "Exercise Tolerance and Cerebral Function after Acute Hemodilution of Polycythemic Mountain Climbers," *The Physiologist* 25 (1982): 327.

9. See F. D. Blume, "Metabolic and Endocrine Changes," in J. B. West and S. Lahiri, eds., *High Altitude and Man* (Washington, D.C.: American Physiological Society, 1984).

10. See J. P. Mordes et al., "High Altitude Pituitary-Thyroid Dysfunction on Mount Everest," *New England Journal of Medicine* 308 (1983): 1135–38.

11. J. S. Milledge et al., "Renin, Angiotensin Converting Enzyme and Aldosterone in Man on Mount Everest," *J. Appl. Physiol.: Respirat. Environ. Exercise Physiol.* 55 (1983): 1109–12.

12. B. D. Townes et al., "Human Cerebral Function at Extreme Altitude," in West and Lahiri, *High Altitude and Man*, pp. 31–36.

13. See R. M. Winslow, "High Altitude Polycythemia," in ibid., pp. 163–72.

14. See R. B. Schoene et al., "Relationship of Hypoxic Ventilatory Response to Exercise Performance on Mount Everest," *J. Appl. Physiol.: Respirat. Environ. Exercise Physiol.* 56 (1984): 1478–83.

Chapter 7

1. From R. Messner, *Everest: Expedition to the Ultimate* (London: Kaye and Ward, 1979), p. 180. This is part of Messner's graphic description of his feelings on reaching the summit at the end of the first ascent (with Habeler) without supplementary oxygen.

2. This transcription of the tape dictated by Glenn Porzak is almost verbatim. The same is true of the debriefing tapes of Kopczynski, Pizzo, and Hackett included in subsequent chapters. In a few places repetition has been omitted.

Chapter 8

1. From Pizzo's debriefing describing his reactions to finding the ice axe above Camp 5.

2. See J. B. West et al., "Pulmonary Gas Exchange on the Summit of Mount Everest," *J. Appl. Physiol.: Respirat. Environ. Exercise Physiol.* 55 (1983): 678–87.

3. See J. B. West et al., "Barometric Pressures at Extreme Altitudes on Mt. Everest: Physiological Significance," *J. Appl. Physiol.: Respirat. Environ. Exercise Physiol.* 54 (1983): 1188–94.

Chapter 9

1. From George Mallory, quoted in Thomas F. Hornbein, *Everest: The West Ridge* (San Francisco: Sierra Club, 1963).

2. Hackett's account was meant for his listeners at Camp 2, not for the world at large. I hope that readers will not be offended by the four-letter words which reflect the release of tension after surviving the solo summit climb. This is not the way that Peter normally talks.

Chapter 10

1. From I. Acosta, *The Naturall and Morall Historie of the East and West Indies* (London: Edward Blount and William Aspley, 1604), p. 148.

Appendix B

1. E. Schneider, "Khumbu Himal Map 1: 50,000," 2d ed. (Vienna: Kartographische Anstalt Freytag-Berndt und Artaria, 1978).

Appendix D

1. F. H. Sarnquist, "Physicians on Mount Everest," *Western Journal of Medicine* 139 (1983): 480–85.

2. See D. A. Sack et al., "Prophylactic Doxycycline for Traveler's Diarrhea," *New England Journal of Medicine* 298 (1978): 758–63; also, R. B. Sack et al., "Prophylactic Doxycycline for Traveler's Diarrhea," *Gastroenterology* 76 (1979): 1368–73.

3. See P. Steele, "Medicine on Mount Everest 1971," *Lancet* 2 (1971): 32–39.

4. See P. H. Hackett, *Mountain Sickness* (New York: American Alpine Club, 1980).

Appendix A
EXPEDITION TEAM AND SHERPAS

Expedition Team (data correct for the time of the expedition)

CLIMBERS

John P. Evans (deputy leader in charge of climbing).
Age 42, married with two children. Academic and professional training in geological sciences. Program Director, Colorado Outward Bound School. Major interests include mountaineering, canoeing, and white-water rafting. Extensive climbing experience in United States, Himalaya, Antarctica, and U.S.S.R. Climbing leader of International Expedition to Everest, 1971.

David P. Jones.
Age 33, single, Canadian nationality. Professional training in physical geography. Extensive climbing experience included 7,800 meters on Makalu in 1974, and 6,800 meters on Manaslu in 1978.

Chris Kopczynski.
Age 29, married, two children. Building contractor. Extensive climbing experience including the Eiger north face, Himalaya including Makalu, also U.S.S.R.

Jeff Lowe.
Age 31, single. Technical consultant to Lowe Alpine Systems. Particularly interested in ice climbing. Extensive climbing experience included south face of Ama Dablam (solo) in 1979, American-U.S.S.R. Palmirs Expedition in 1974, and American Karakorum Latok 1 Expedition, Pakistan, in 1978.

Glenn E. Porzak.
Age 33, married, two children. Attorney. Law degree from University of Colorado. Extensive climbing experience including over 30 ascents in the European Alps, and expeditions to Mt. Aconcagua, Hindu Kush, Manaslu, and Cordilleira Blanca. Chairman of the Expeditions Committee of the American Alpine Club.

EVEREST

Michael H. Weis.
Age 31, single. Self-employed mountain guide with 11 years experience. Climbing experience includes North America, two expeditions to South America, French Alps.

CLIMBING SCIENTISTS

Steven Boyer.
Age 35, single. M.D. from University of Colorado. Emergency room physician, University of Oregon Medical Center. Marathon runner, including Pike's Peak marathon in 1977. Competitive cross-country skier. Extensive climbing experience in North America, Ecuador, Peru, New Zealand, and Antarctica.

David J. Graber.
Age 29, married. M.D. from Baylor University, 1978. Emergency room physician, Valley Medical Center, Fresno, California. Extensive climbing experience in North America, Iran, Nepal. Led a party of 6 climbers to the Garhwal Himalaya. Extensive experience as an expedition physician.

Peter H. Hackett.
Age 33, single. M.D. from University of Illinois. Medical director, Himalayan Rescue Association, Pheriche. Worked as emergency room physician in Bishop, California. Extensive experience on medical problems of high altitude, and author of a book on this subject. Climbing experience in Nepal includes Island Peak, Lobuya Peak, and Baruntse.

Christopher J. Pizzo.
Age 32, single. M.D. from Indiana University. Main research interest immunopathology. Competitive marathon runner, including Pike's Peak marathon in 1979. Extensive climbing experience in North and South America, India, Nepal, U.S.S.R. First American ascent of Pik Kommunizma.

Frank H. Sarnquist.
Age 39, married, one child. M.D. from University of California, San Francisco. Assistant professor of anesthesia, Stanford University Medical School. Extensive climbing experience in North America, South America, and Australia. Has been physician to several climbing expeditions.

Robert B. Schoene.
Age 34, married, two children. M.D. from Columbia College of Physicians and Surgeons. Faculty member, Division of Respiratory Diseases, Department of Medicine, University of Washington, Seattle. Several publications in high-altitude medicine. Competitive marathon runner. Climbing experience mainly in North America.

SCIENTISTS

F. Duane Blume (deputy leader in charge of logistics and finance).
Age 48, married, nine children. Ph.D. from University of California, Berkeley. Past assistant director of the University of California, White Mountain High Altitude Research Station, Bishop, California. Chairman of the Department of Biology, California State

College, Bakersfield. A member of the International Everest Expedition in 1971 where he was responsible for the oxygen equipment. Several publications on metabolism at high altitude.

Sukhamay Lahiri.
Age 48, married, no children. Born West Bengal, India. D.Phil. from Oxford University, U.K., 1959. Associate professor of physiology, University of Pennsylvania. Was a physiologist on the Himalayan Scientific and Mountaineering Expedition, 1960–61, scientific leader of the Himalayan Scientific and Schoolhouse Expedition, 1964, and leader of a physiological expedition to the Andes, 1969–70. Numerous scientific articles on high-altitude physiology.

Karl H. Maret.
Age 33, married, no children. Canadian citizen. M.E. in biomedical engineering, and M.D. from University of Toronto. Participated in the Mt. Logan High Altitude Physiology Expedition of 1975. Employed by the Fashioners of Manas, Inc., a group interested in holistic health.

James S. Milledge.
Age 51, married, two children. British nationality. M.D. from University of Birmingham. Consultant physician, Northwick Park Hospital, London; scientific staff member, British Medical Research Council. Was a member of the Himalayan Scientific and Mountaineering Expedition, 1960–61, 2nd Himalayan Schoolhouse Expedition of 1964, and a physiological expedition to the Sola Khumbu in 1970. Many publications in the area of high-altitude physiology. Considerable climbing experience including first ascent of Puma Dablam, Nepal.

Richard M. Peters, Jr.
Age 25, single. B.A. from Stanford University. Waiting to enter UCSD Medical School. Extensive construction experience, carpentry, electrical, machine shop. Excellent skier.

Michele Samaja.
Age 30, married, no children. Italian citizen. Ph.D. from University of Milan. Senior investigator in the Department of Biological Chemistry, Department of Medicine, University of Milan. Took part in an Italian Scientific expedition to the Everest Base Camp in 1976. Has published extensively on blood physiology. Experienced rock climber in the Italian Dolomites.

John B. West (expedition leader).
Age 52, married, two children. M.D. and D.Sc. from University of Adelaide; Ph.D. from University of London. Professor of medicine and physiology, University of California, San Diego. Was a physiologist on the Himalayan Scientific and Mountaineering Expedition, 1960–61. Particular interests are respiratory, high-altitude, and space physiology. Extensive publications in these areas.

Robert M. Winslow.
Age 40, married, two children. M.D. from Johns Hopkins University. Member of the

scientific staff, Centers for Disease Control, Atlanta. Led a research team studying high-altitude physiology in the Peruvian Andes. Extensive list of publications on hemoglobin and its physiology, particularly the effects of high altitude.

BASE CAMP MANAGER

Rodney A. Korich.
Age 34, single. Extensive climbing and base camp manager experience in Nepal, including Makalu in 1974 and 1977, and Dhaulagiri, 1980. Also was on Aconcagua, Argentina.

LIAISON OFFICERS

Yogendra Thapa, police officer, Kathmandu.
Mingma Gyelgen Sherpa, physician, Terhathum.

HIGH-ALTITUDE SHERPAS

Sonam Girme, 45, (sirdar), Namche Bazar; Young Tenzing, 31, Namche Bazar; Nuru Jangbo, 27, Thyangboche; Sungdare, 27, Thyangboche; Pasang Tenzing, 51, Kudu; Lhakpa Gyalu, 45, Namche Bazar; Pasang Gyaljen, 26, Phortse; Ang Nuwu, 33, Khumjung; Nima Tshering, 45, Khumjung; Dorje, 23, Khumjung; Pemba Nuru, 26, Khunde; Ang Jangbo, 21, Phortse; Ang Lhakpa, 23, Khunde; Ang Nima, 22, Khunde; Pasang Sona, 33, Khumjung; Gyaljen, 30, Phortse; Ang Phurba, 22, Thame; Ang Tshering, 27, Thame; Kilu Temba, 21, Thame; Ang Kami, 36, Thame; Ang Pasang, 31, Thame; Ang Pemba, 33, Thomde; Pasang Dawa, 41, Khunde; Pasang Sona, 46, Khunde; Ang Nima, 39, Namche; Lhakpa Temba, 26, Ghat; Phuru, 25, Angripan; Nima Kancha, 29, Jarok; Chewang, 28, Solu; Namgyal, 21, Namche Bazar; Jangbu, 32, Chermang Dingma; Dawa Gyaljen, 32, Chermang Dingma; Ang Tshering, 29, Thame; Sonam Temba, 43, Thado Kosi; Phurba Kitar, 31, Nazi Pangdok; Nima Rita, 41, Phortse; Kancha Tamang, 30, Dada Kharka; Kancha, 41 (high-altitude cook), Khunde; Ang Pema, 49 (Base Camp cook), Khunde; Mingma Tamang, 25 (Base Camp kitchen boy), Kerong Solu; Dendi, 27 (Base Camp kitchen boy), Solu; Kancha, 26 (mail runner), Solu.

Appendix B
DIARY OF EVENTS AND TABLE OF CAMPS

1960–61	Himalayan Scientific and Mountaineering Expedition. Considerably influenced the design of the present expedition. Three members—Lahiri, Milledge, and West—were members of both expeditions.
September 1974	Jim Milledge and I discuss the possibility of doing more physiological measurements at high altitudes in the Himalaya.
January 20, 1976	Application for a research contract sent to National Heart, Lung and Blood Institute to support physiological research on the 1977 New Zealand Everest expedition. Plan fell through. Nevertheless, valuable experience was obtained in testing the Medilog recorder, particularly when Chris Chandler, M.D., took it to the Everest summit during the American Bicentennial expedition of 1976.
1977	Duane Blume and I begin planning a dedicated physiological expedition to Everest. John Evans chosen as climbing leader.
January 10, 1978	Official application to the Ministry of Tourism in Nepal.
June 25	Official period of permission received for postmonsoon period, 1981.
October 11	Grant application submitted to National Institutes of Health to begin design and construction of special scientific equipment for the expedition.
July 1979	Grant funded. Work on the equipment begins.
1979–80	Expedition team chosen.
March 1980	Base Camp laboratory hut, and scientific tent for Camp 5 tested on the summit of Mammoth Mountain, altitude 3,350 meters (11,000 feet).
January 1981	Ten tons of equipment and food shipped from Los Angeles to Calcutta en route for Kathmandu.
April–May	Equipment carried in to Sola Khumbu area to await arrival of expedition.

163

EVEREST

May	Expedition members come to University of California, San Diego, for baseline testing.
July 25	Blume, Evans, Peters, and I fly from Seattle. (Most of the rest of the expedition leave one week later.)
August 6	Expedition moves from Kathmandu to Dolalghat by bus.
August 8	We begin trek into Base Camp.
August 30	Base Camp established at the head of the Khumbu Glacier, altitude 5,400 meters (17,700 feet).
September 1	5 A.M. Boyer, Kopczynski, Pizzo, and Porzak start on finding a route through the icefall.
September 3	Boyer and Kopczynski reach suitable site for Camp 1.
September 5	Heavy snowfall prevents further work in the icefall until September 12.
September 13	Camp 1 established at 5,950 meters (19,500 feet). Sherpas begin carrying loads through the icefall.
September 15	Camp 2 established in the Western Cwm at 6,300 meters (20,700 feet).
September 24	Camp 3 established on the southwest buttress of Everest at 7,250 meters (23,800 feet). Science laboratory hut set up at Camp 2, though the research program not going full speed ahead until October 4.
September 27–29	Severe storm with gale force winds at Camp 2.
October 5	Camp 4 established at approximately 7,500 meters (24,500 feet).
October 11	Jones, Kopczynski, and Pizzo establish Camp 5 60 meters above the South Col at an altitude of 8,050 meters (26,400 feet). High winds force their return to Camp 2 on October 14.
October 12	Pizzo measures barometric pressure at Camp 5, and takes a series of alveolar gas samples on Jones, Kopczynski, and himself.
October 15	Hackett, Porzak, and Thapa reach Camp 5 hoping to make a summit attempt. High winds force them to abandon this, and they return to Camp 2 on October 17.
October 20	Kopczynski and Weis with sherpas arrive at Camp 5 but find that only one tent has survived the storms. Mike goes down, leaving Kop and Sungdare for a summit bid.
October 21	Kopczynski and Sungdare leave Camp 5 at 7 A.M. and reach the summit at 11:20 A.M. They use Hornbein oxygen equipment. Kop unable to find the Camp 5 science equipment, and no measurements were made.
October 23	Hackett, Pizzo, Nuru Jangbo, and Young Tenzing reach Camp 5, and prepare the science equipment.
October 24	Pizzo and Young Tenzing leave Camp 5 at 6:30 A.M., and reach the summit at 12:30 P.M. Chris wears Medilog recorder, and measures maximal exercise ventilation en route to the summit. He measures

164

barometric pressure and temperature on the summit, and takes alveolar gas samples. On the way down he measures resting ventilation at an altitude of 8,400 meters (27,600 feet) while waiting for Hackett to return.

Hackett and Nuru Jangbo set out for the summit at about 7:30 A.M. but Nuru Jangbo returns to Camp 5. Hackett gives up hope of reaching summit, but walks up the mountain to meet Pizzo and Young Tenzing as they descend. The three meet at 2 P.M. below the South Summit, and Hackett decides to make a solo summit attempt. He summits at 4 P.M. while Pizzo waits for him at the old Camp 6 site (8,400 meters, 27,600 feet). Hackett falls while negotiating the Hillary Step on the way down, but recovers to join Pizzo at 6 P.M. They descend in the dark to Camp 5, reaching it at 8 P.M.

October 25	Pizzo and Hackett measure barometric pressure, and take alveolar gas and venous blood samples from each other at Camp 5. They then descend to Camp 2.
October 26	Another storm at Camp 2.
October 27	Remaining climbers and scientists return from Camp 2 to Base Camp. Mountain cleared of all equipment except for damaged tents at Camp 5 and some fixed ropes on the headwall.
October 31	Base Camp cleared and vacated.

EXPEDITION CAMPS

		Date established	Altitude		Evidence for altitude	Barometric pressure (mmHg)
	Location		meters	feet		
Base Camp	Foot of Khumbu ice fall	8/30/81	5,400	17,700	Schneider map[1]	398–402
Camp 1	Top of ice fall	9/13/81	5,950	19,500	Barometric pressure	366
Camp 2	Western Cwm	9/15/81	6,300	20,700	Pressure and map	350–352
Camp 3	Headwall	9/24/81	7,250	23,800	Barometric pressure	309
Camp 4	Headwall	10/5/81	7,500	24,500	Estimated	not measured
Camp 5	Just above South Col	10/11/81	8,050	26,400	Visual estimate above South Col	280–285
Summit		(ascents) 10/21/81 10/24/81	8,848	29,028	Schneider map[1] and other authorities	250–253

Appendix C

LIST OF SCIENTIFIC ARTICLES FROM THE EXPEDITION

Blume, F. D. Metabolic and endocrine changes. In *High Altitude and Man*, ed. J. B. West and S. Lahiri. Washington, D.C.: American Physiological Society, 1984.

Blume, F. D., S. J. Boyer, L. E. Braverman, A. Cohen, J. Dirkse, and J. P. Mordes. Impaired osmoregulation at extreme altitude. *J. Amer. Med. Assoc.* 252 (1984): 524–526.

Boyer, S. J., and F. D. Blume. Weight loss and changes in body composition at high altitude. *J. Appl. Physiol.* 57 (1984): 1580–85.

Hackett, P. H., F. H. Sarnquist, and R. B. Schoene. Hemodilution of polycythemic mountaineers: effect on exercise and mental function. Unpublished paper.

Hackett, P. H., R. B. Schoene, R. M. Winslow, R. M. Peters, Jr., and J. B. West. Acetazolamide and exercise in sojourners to 6,300 meters. *Medicine and Science in Sports and Exercise*. In press.

Karliner, J. S., F. H. Sarnquist, D. J. Graber, R. M. Peters, Jr., and J. B. West. The electrocardiogram at extreme altitude: experience on Mt. Everest. *Amer. Heart J.* In press.

Lahiri, S. Human adaptation to high altitude: lessons from Sherpa physiology. In *Human Genetics and Human Adaptation*, ed. A. Basu and K. C. Malhotra. Calcutta, Indian Statistical Institute, 1984.

———. Respiratory control in Andean and Himalayan high altitude natives. In *High Altitude and Man*, ed. J. B. West and S. Lahiri. Washington, D.C.: American Physiological Society, 1984.

———. Role of peripheral chemoreflex in breathing pattern during sleep at high altitude. In *Hypoxia, Exercise and Altitude*, ed. John R. Sutton, Charles S. Houston, and Norman L. Jones. New York: Alan R. Liss, 1983.

Lahiri, S., K. Maret, and M. G. Sherpa. Dependence of high altitude sleep apnea on ventilatory sensitivity to hypoxia. *Respir. Physiol.* 52 (1983): 281–301.

Lahiri, S., K. Maret, M. G. Sherpa, and R. M. Peters, Jr. Sleep and periodic breathing at high altitude: Sherpa natives vs. sojourners. In *High Altitude and Man*, ed. J. B. West and S. Lahiri. Washington, D.C.: American Physiological Society, 1984.

Maret, K. H. Expedition to Mt. Everest, 1981: technical aspects. In *Hypoxia: Man at Altitude*, ed. J. R. Sutton, N. L. Jones, and C. S. Houston. New York: Thieme-Stratton, 1982.

Maret, K. H., J. O. Billups, R. M. Peters, Jr., and J. B. West. Automatic mechanical alveolar gas sampler for multiple sample collection in the field. *J. Appl. Physiol.: Respirat. Environ. Exercise Physiol.* 56 (1984): 1435–38.

Milledge, J. S. Renin-aldosterone system. In *High Altitude and Man*, ed. J. B. West and S. Lahiri. Washington, D.C.: American Physiological Society, 1984.

Milledge, J. S., D. M. Catley, F. D. Blume, and J. B. West. Renin, angiotensin converting enzyme and aldosterone in man on Mount Everest. *J. Appl. Physiol.: Respirat. Environ. Exercise Physiol.* 55 (1983): 1109–12.

Mordes, J. P., F. D. Blume, S. Boyer, M.-R. Zheng, and L. E. Braverman. High altitude pituitary-thyroid dysfunction on Mount Everest. *New England Journal of Medicine*. 308 (1983): 1135–38.

Sarnquist, F. H. Physicians on Mount Everest. *West. J. Med.* 139 (1983): 480–85.

Schoene, R. B. Hypoxic chemosensitivity and ventilation. In *High Altitude and Man*, ed. J. B. West and S. Lahiri. Washington, D.C.: American Physiological Society, 1984.

———. Science on high: the 1981 American Medical Research Expedition to Everest. *Respir. Care.* 27 (1982): 1519–24.

Schoene, R. B., S. Lahiri, P. H. Hackett, R. M. Peters, Jr., J. S. Milledge, C. J. Pizzo, F. H. Sarnquist, S. J. Boyer, D. J. Graber, K. H. Maret, and J. B. West. Relationship of hypoxic ventilatory response to exercise performance on Mount Everest. *J. Appl. Physiol.: Respirat. Environ. Exercise Physiol.* 56 (1984): 1478–83.

Townes, B. D., T. F. Hornbein, R. B. Schoene, F. H. Sarnquist, and I. Grant. Human cerebral function at extreme altitude. In *High Altitude and Man*, ed. J. B. West and S. Lahiri. Washington, D.C.: American Physiological Society, 1984.

West, J. B. American Medical Research Expedition to Everest: a study of man during extreme hypoxia. In *Hypoxia, Exercise, and Altitude*, ed. by John R. Sutton, Charles S. Houston, and Norman L. Jones. Progress in Clinical and Biological Research, volume 136. New York: Alan R. Liss, 1983.

———. American Medical Research Expedition to Everest, 1981. *Himalayan Journal*. 39 (1983): 19–25.

———. American Medical Research Expedition to Everest, 1981. *The Physiologist*. 25 (1982): 36–38.

———. American Medical Research Expedition to Everest, 1981. *Seminars in Respiratory Medicine*. 5 (1983): 126–28.

————. Climbing Mt. Everest without oxygen: an analysis of maximal exercise during extreme hypoxia. *Resp. Physiol.* 52 (1983): 265–79.

————. Human physiology at extreme altitudes on Mount Everest. *Science.* 223 (February 24, 1984): 784–88.

————. Lessons learned on the mountain. *Bulletin, American College of Surgeons* 68 (1983): 9–14.

————. Man at extreme altitude. *J. Appl. Physiol.: Respirat. Environ. Exercise Physiol.* 52 (1982): 1393–99.

————. Man on the summit of Mount Everest. In *High Altitude and Man*, ed. J. B. West and S. Lahiri. Washington, D.C.: American Physiological Society, 1984.

————. "Oxygenless" climbs and barometric pressure. *American Alpine Journal.* 58 (1984): 126–32.

————. Pulmonary gas transfer. *Respiration and Circulation.* 53 (1983): 511–18.

————. Science on Everest, 1981. In *Hypoxia: Man at Altitude*, ed. J. R. Sutton, N. L. Jones, and C. S. Houston. New York: Thieme-Stratton, 1982.

West, J. B., S. J. Boyer, D. J. Graber, P. H. Hackett, K. H. Maret, J. S. Milledge, R. M. Peters, Jr., C. J. Pizzo, M. Samaja, F. H. Sarnquist, R. B. Schoene, and R. M. Winslow. Maximal exercise at extreme altitudes on Mount Everest. *J. Appl. Physiol.: Respirat. Environ. Exercise Physiol.* 55 (1983): 688–98.

West, J. B., and J. P. Evans. American Medical Research Expedition to Everest. *American Alpine Journal.* 24 (1982): 53–68.

West, J. B., P. H. Hackett, K. H. Maret, J. S. Milledge, R. M. Peters, Jr., C. J. Pizzo, and R. M. Winslow. Human physiology on the summit of Mount Everest. *Trans. Assn. Amer. Phys.* 95 (1982): 63–70.

————. Pulmonary gas exchange on the summit of Mount Everest. *J. Appl. Physiol.: Respirat. Environ. Exercise Physiol.* 55 (1983): 678–87.

West, J. B., P. H. Hackett, K. H. Maret, R. M. Peters, Jr., C. J. Pizzo, and R. M. Winslow. Hypoxia at extreme altitude. *Bull. europ. Physiopath. resp.* 18, suppl. 4 (1982): 21–28.

West, J. B., S. Lahiri, K. H. Maret, R. M. Peters, Jr., and C. J. Pizzo. Barometric pressures at extreme altitudes on Mt. Everest: physiological significance. *J. Appl. Physiol.: Respirat. Environ. Exercise Physiol.* 54: 1188–94, 1983.

Winslow, R. M. Red cell function at extreme altitude. In *High Altitude and Man*, ed. J. B. West and S. Lahiri. Washington, D.C.: American Physiological Society, 1984.

Winslow, R. M., and M. Samaja. Red cell function on Mount Everest. *Bull. europ. Physiopath. resp.* 18, suppl. 4 (1982): 35–38.

Winslow, R. M., M. Samaja, and J. B. West. Red cell function at extreme altitude on Mount Everest. *J. Appl. Physiol.: Respirat. Environ. Exercise Physiol.* 56 (1984): 109–16.

Appendix D
MEDICAL PROBLEMS
by Frank H. Sarnquist, M.D.

This brief account has been abstracted from a longer article.[1] Dr. Frank Sarnquist was responsible for the medical aspects of the expedition, including prevention and treatment of disease. We always maintained a clear distinction between this aspect of the expedition and the medical research objectives.

PREPARATIONS

Prior to the expedition each member had a complete medical examination. This was done when the members met at the University of California, San Diego, in May 1981 for the baseline physiology tests.

A full medical history was taken, and each member filled out a detailed questionnaire. This was followed by a complete physical examination including detailed dental and eye examinations. Laboratory tests included blood type, complete blood count, chest X-ray, 12-lead electrocardiogram, urinalysis, and skin test for tuberculosis.

In addition, all members were advised to have poliomyelitis, tetanus, diphtheria, and typhoid immunizations. Gamma globulin (2 cc. intramuscularly) was given just prior to leaving the United States as prophylaxis against hepatitis. Antimalarial tablets were not recommended.

Vibramycin (doxycycline) 250 mg. orally each day was made available for the prophylaxis of diarrhea. However, this was optional. Members were also given information on the use of the first aid kit.

The contents of personal first aid kits were as follows: adhesive tape, Bandaids, aspirin, aspirin with codeine (30 mg.), Lomotil (diphenoxylate with atropine), Dalmane (15 mg.) (flurazepam), Ornade (cold tablet), Cepacol throat lozenges, Dexedrine (5 mg.) (dextroamphetamine), multi-vitamins, safety pins, elastic bandages, Moleskin, Vibramycin (doxycycline) (only for those who elected to take it prophylactically), instruction sheet.

In addition, every member was encouraged to come to the mountain as physically fit as possible, and most had an exercise program such as daily running for several months before the expedition.

EVEREST

TREK TO BASE CAMP

Here we had a careful program of simple public health measures aimed primarily at assuring the purity of food and water. This included the complete avoidance in any form of untreated water, and ingestion of only thoroughly cooked food (or unbroken fruits and vegetables that could be peeled and washed in treated water). In addition, we educated and supervised our kitchen sherpas on hand washing, food and water handling, and washing of dishes. All the sherpas who worked in the kitchen received a single oral dose of Vermox (mebendazole) to rid them of intestinal parasites.

An important element was a water purification system (donated by the Wal-Bro Company of Ann Arbor, Michigan), which provided an immediate supply of potable cold water, a luxury in a country where virtually all water is polluted. This system uses an ion exchange resin to iodinate water. It includes small purifiers for each member to treat drinking water along the trail, and large purifiers that provided the quantity of water needed for cooking, hand washing, and dish washing for several dozen people.

Doxycycline, along with evidence of its efficacy and toxicity, was offered to all expedition members, but the decision to take the drug was optional. About half the members took the drug, and these members apparently had fewer attacks of diarrhea, and those attacks which did occur were shorter in duration. These results are similar to those obtained in more rigorous studies of the effectiveness of tetracyclines in preventing and ameliorating "turista."[2]

In all diarrhea cases, sufferers were urged to tolerate the disease for a day, which in most cases was adequate time for spontaneous recovery. If the condition persisted, treatment was begun with Flagyl (metronidazole) if *giardia lamblia* was suspected as the causative agent (diarrhea plus bloating and foul smelling belching), or Bactrim DS (trimethoprim and sulfamethaxazole) if the diarrhea was complicated by fever and toxic symptoms. In these cases Lomotil (diphenoxylate and atropine) was also used for symptomatic relief. Three cases required more than one course of treatment.

A flulike syndrome struck several members during the approach, and was treated symptomatically. Cutters Insect Repellant appeared to be an effective leech repellant when used regularly. One infected leech bite would not heal despite antibiotics and intensive local wound care, and made it impossible for the affected sherpa to wear boots, preventing him from working on the mountain.

ON THE MOUNTAIN

The pattern of health problems changed after reaching Base Camp. Leeches and polluted water were below us, and were replaced by the problems of living in the cold, dry, oxygen-poor air of Mt. Everest. From Base Camp on, the preventative medicine program switched emphasis from public health measures to careful attention to three personal health goals: to keep the expedition members abundantly hydrated, well fed, and adequately rested. We feel that the outstanding physical performance of the expedition members, two of whom climbed the final 800 vertical meters on Mt. Everest in under 5 hours, attested to the success of this program. In addition, the enormous effort made by everyone to remain hydrated, nourished, and rested contributed to the relative paucity of medical problems encountered.

Even these measures did not obviate all problems. Sore throat, runny nose, and dry, chronic cough affected every member of the expedition. Occasionally these symptoms were disabling, but generally only annoying. "Colds" were treated with a combination of medically unproven maneuvers, including rest, juice, alcohol, vitamin C, cough drops, antihistamines, aspirin, and "cold" tablets. In cases accompanied by fever, muscle pain, purulent sputum, or enlarged lymph glands, an antibiotic (usually ampicillin) was used.

Infections distant from the respiratory tract were the next most prevalent problem. Nearly every accidental wound, no matter how small, suppurated (became pussy) for a period of time, and healed slowly. Several wounds, particularly of the hands, but including one leech bite, did not heal at all until the patient went to lower altitude. The most frightening infection was an olecranon bursitis (inflammation of tissue around the elbow), which rapidly progressed to a cellulitis (inflammation of surrounding tissue) involving the entire arm from wrist to shoulder. Resistant to rest, heat, and oral antibiotics, the infection was finally brought under control by descent to lower elevation, and intravenous cephalosporin (an antibiotic).

Several expedition members suffered a syndrome of sore throat, mild fever, tender neck lymph glands, and malaise. We knew that an epidemic of a "glandular feverlike" illness, later identified as caused by an adenovirus, greatly weakened a previous Mt. Everest expedition.[3] The exact nature and cause of this problem on our trip was not identified, and recovery was spontaneous with return to lower altitudes.

In all, 40 percent of the members of our expedition suffered significant infections (not including the universal upper respiratory tract troubles). The reason for this high incidence of infection in otherwise fit individuals is unclear. Whether the chronic hypoxic state depresses the immune response, or whether the problem is hypoxic interference with wound healing combined with marginal personal hygiene, or some other factor altogether, is a question to be answered in the future.

The most intriguing medical problems were the various manifestations of acute mountain sickness (AMS). This term encompasses a variety of symptoms that occur when sea-level residents ascend to higher elevations. Mild symptoms include headache, lethargy, insomnia, and anorexia (loss of appetite). If the individual does not rest or descend to a lower altitude, these symptoms can progress to shortness of breath, painful nonproductive cough, peripheral edema, cyanosis, nausea, weakness, and a mental state of indifference. In its most severe form, AMS progresses to pulmonary and cerebral edema, unconsciousness, severe arterial desaturation, and death.[4]

AMS can usually be avoided by a gradual ascent. The maxim is: ascend slowly, and if you feel poorly or become ill, descend quickly. Our expedition was careful to ascend at a rate comfortable for all its members, but despite our care, two members and one visitor to the expedition developed high-altitude pulmonary edema (HAPE).

The variable presentation of HAPE was impressively demonstrated during our expedition. The visitor to the expedition, age 25, felt unwell on his initial ascent to high altitude. He descended and then reascended to Base Camp (5,400 meters, 17,700 feet), and spent nine days there feeling reasonably well. On his tenth night at this altitude he awoke at night severely short of breath, coughing, and with rales (bubbling sounds heard with the stethoscope) throughout both lung fields. Fortunately he was sharing a tent with a chest physician who quickly diagnosed HAPE, made the patient comfortable sitting up, and administered oxygen by face mask. By the morning the ill visitor was able to walk with assistance, and he descended to a lower altitude where he made an uneventful recovery.

One of the expedition's most powerful athletes developed mild HAPE after strenuous climbing with a heavy backpack to Camp 3 (7,250 meters, 23,800 feet). The HAPE rapidly cleared with descent, and he later reascended to 8,050 meters (26,400 feet) using supplementary oxygen via a mask, and spent several nights at 7,500 meters (24,600 feet) without difficulty. After a rest at lower altitude he again climbed high on the mountain, but this time he ascended to Camp 4 (7,500 meters, 24,500 feet) with a sizable pack and no supplementary oxygen. He became ill, and returned to Camp 2 complaining of severe postural dyspnea (shortness of breath on lying down), which he characterized as "a feeling of drowning in tracheal secretions [he is a physician] whenever I lie down." It was noticeable that he was able to make good speed down the glacier, but even the smallest uphill section of terrain was a terrible strain, and he became visibly cyanotic (skin became blue) with the effort. When he arrived at Base Camp his arterial oxygen saturation was measured using the oximeter, and found to be 70 percent. Although this was low, the more striking finding was a profound drop to 50 percent saturation with very mild exercise. This climber too recovered quickly at Base Camp.

The other case of HAPE occurred in an expedition member who was asthmatic and had considerable difficulty with his airway disease during the climb. Nevertheless, he ascended to Camp 4 (7,500 meters, 24,500 feet), and played a major role in establishing camps 3 and 4. On his return from the upper camps he had a combination of bronchitis, asthma, and chest congestion. With the resolution of his first two problems with antibiotics and rest, it was apparent that he had a significant component of pulmonary edema that cleared only after descent to Base Camp and oxygen administration for two days. We saw no evidence of cerebral edema in any of our members.

Severe peripheral cold injury (frostbite) has been a major cause of morbidity during previous attempts to climb Mt. Everest. Our group suffered no frostbite, and we feel that our attention to personal health measures, and our excellent insulating clothing and boots protected us. Although much of our gear was the current version of traditional designs and materials, the use of three recently developed materials is worth noting. All the high-altitude climbers wore windproof suits made of a teflon-nylon laminate. The expanded teflon membrane (Goretex) is bonded to the nylon and to the fabric to make a material that is totally windproof without being excessively heavy or impermeable to water vapor generated by the body. Goretex was also used as a covering in our sleeping bags, which were filled with goose down.

Our boots (Koflach) were fashioned of a nylonlike material that is durable and extremely lightweight. Although this material does not have exceptional insulating properties, it never becomes wet or frozen, and its rigidity protects the feet from pressure caused by straps used to secure crampons. These boots were comfortable and entirely satisfactory.

Insulating clothing fashioned of a furlike synthetic pile fabric was widely used. This pile fabric is soft, nonirritating, lightweight, and warm. It does not absorb moisture, and thus retains its insulating properties when wet, and it dries quickly. It largely replaced wool on our expedition as the preferred fabric for underwear, sweaters, and trousers.

Our diet was based on locally available fresh food. Marvelous potatoes and winter vegetables are grown only a few days' walk from Base Camp, and are available in limited quantities in the autumn. Rice and lentils, as well as occasional fruits, were also available. We perhaps set a world's altitude record by sprouting several kinds of seeds and beans at Camp 2 (6,300 meters, 20,700 feet). We supplemented the locally available foods with a large and varied selection of preserved foods brought from the U.S., including canned ham, tuna, crabmeat, and salmon, breakfast cereals, candy, cookies, dried fruits and meats. We used very little freeze-dried food as previous experiences had convinced us that food preserved in this manner was unsatisfying and often tasteless at altitude.

Little alcohol was included in our rations, and this scarcity seemed to cause no great hardship. In the lowlands moderate amounts of excellent Nepalese beer were consumed when it was available. No one smoked cigarettes above Base Camp in spite of Finch's remarkable claim in 1922 that smoking reduced the feeling of breathlessness at 25,500 feet on Everest. A variety of food supplements and vitamins were used by individual members of the expedition, without any obvious advantages or drawbacks.

Appendix E

GRANTS AND BENEFACTORS

MAJOR GRANTS TO THE EXPEDITION

National Institutes of Health Grant, "Human Respiratory Function at Extreme Altitudes" (principal investigator, West), $181,566.

National Institutes of Health Grant, "Altered Respiratory Control in Chronic Hypoxemia" (Lahiri), $73,228.

U.S. Army Research and Development Command Contract, "Factors Determining Tolerance to High Altitude" (West), $44,888.

Les Laboratoires Servier (Paris), "Effects of Almitrine on Ventilation at High Altitude" (West), $38,800.

National Geographic Society (West), $35,000.

National Science Foundation Grant, "Metabolic and Endocrine Function at Extreme Altitudes" (Blume), $31,212.

National Institutes of Health Contract, "Respiratory Function at Extreme Altitude" (West), $30,455.

American Lung Association (Sarnquist), $15,310.

UCSD Chancellor's Associates (West), $5,000.

UCSD Academic Senate Committee on Research (West), $3,160.

Total grants: $458,619

BENEFACTORS

We wish to thank the following donors who made the expedition possible.

FOOD

American Popcorn Company, ARDA, Betty Crocker, Celestial Seasonings Herb Tea, CPC International, Del Monte, Foremost McKesson Foods, G. A. Hormel & Co., General Mills, General Nutrition Corp., Golden Grain Macaroni Company, Goodmark Foods, Gookinaid ERG, Gregg Foods, Hickory Farms, H. J. Heinz Co., Jeno's, Joyva Corporation, Kikkoman Intern., Inc., Knorr Swiss, Krusteaz, Liberty Orchards Co. Inc., Maruchan Inc., McIlhenny Co., M&M/Mars, Mother's Cake and Cookie Company, Nalley's Fine Foods, Pacific Pearl Seafood, Peter Pan Seafoods, Peter Paul Cadbury, Plumrose, Quaker Oats, Reynolds Aluminum, RJR Foods, Romanoff Caviar Co., Roman Meal Co., Ross Laboratories, Sanna Division (Beatrice Foods), Silver State Foods, Societe Candy Co., Specialty Seafoods, Stone-Wheat (Orowheat), Sunny Jim, The East Asiatic Company-Danola, The Smithfield Ham & Products Co. Inc., T. M. Duche Nut Company, Tom's Foods, Wallis Energy Paks, Ward Johnston Inc., Wee-Pak, Weetabix Ltd., Wilbur Ellis Co., Wm. Underwood Co.

CLIMBING EQUIPMENT

Alpine Map Co., Alpine Research Inc., Camp 7, Forrest Mountaineering Ltd., Frostline Kits, Kelty Pack Inc., Liberty Organization Inc., Lowe Alpine Systems, Mountain Safety Research, Robert C. Maillot/Interalp-Camp, Robbins Mountaingear & Mountainwear, Seattle Manufacturing Corp., Sherpa, Inc., Sierra Designs, The Coleman Company, Inc., The Hardware Store of Evergreen, The North Face, True Temper Corporation, Wonder Corporation of America.

CLOTHING

Arthur Kahn Company, Banana Equipment, Bausch & Lomb, B.R.S., Inc. (Nike), Damart Thermawear, Eddie Bauer, Factory Surplus, Inter Shoes of America, Manudieci Milano, Marmot Mountain Works Ltd., Midwest Feather & Down Company, Scandia Trading Company, Volvo of America Corporation, Wigwam Mills Inc., W. L. Gore & Associates.

SCIENTIFIC EQUIPMENT

Airesearch Manufacturing Company of California, American Klegecell Corp., American Optical, ANCO Engineers, Beckman Instruments Inc., Becton Dickinson Corporation, Bird Electronics, Bobadilla Cases, Boehringer Laboratories, Calmont Engineering and Electronics Corp., Continental Forest Industries, Crystalloid Electronics, Domtar Packaging, Doug Deeds Design Associates, Dow Chemical Corporation, E. I. Dupont Inc., Envi Record Inc., Gas Tech Inc., General Diagnostics, General Electric Corp./Mobile Communications Division, Glad Division-Union Carbide, Golden Engineering, Gould Inc./Automotive Battery Division, Gould Inc./Instruments Division, Hans Rudolph, Inc., Hansen Weather Port Corp., Hewlett-Packard Inc., Hydro Flame Corporation, InspirAir Corp., Kaysam Corporation of America, Lantuck Mills, Lumiscope Co. Inc., Mammoth Mountain Ski Area, Matheson Corp., Meriam Instrument, Miles Laboratories Inc., Mittry Interiors, National Semiconductor, Oxford Medilog Inc., Panasonic Corporation/Matsushita Electric Co., Philips Business Systems Inc., Physio-Control Corp., P. K. Morgan Ltd., Powertec, Inc., Progressive Yacht Hardware Inc., Quantum Instruments, Revue Thommen Ltd., Siemens

Corporation of America, Sierracin/Western Thermidor, Stihl Inc., Therm'x Corp., Topax Electronics, Transpo Electronics, Inc., VBA Cryogenics, Worthington Cylinders.

MEDICAL SUPPLIES

Ambu-International, American Optical Company, Argon Medical Corp., Baxter-Travenol Laboratories, Boehringer Ingelheim Ltd., Bristol Laboratories, Cutter Laboratories, Eli Lilly and Company, Endo Laboratories, Hewlett-Packard Company, Hoffman-La Roche Inc., Johnson and Johnson, Jones Ambulance Service, Lederle Laboratories, Marion Laboratories Inc., McNeil Med Spec, Merrell-National Laboratories, Mid Valley Surgical Supply, Narco Air Shields, Passmore Dental, Reed & Carnick, Schering Corporation, Searle, Siemens-Elema, Smith, Klein and French, Surgikos, The Upjohn Company, Welch-Allyn, Westwood Pharmaceuticals Inc., Wilbur Ellis Company, William H. Rorer Inc., Winthrop Laboratories, Wyeth Laboratories.

CASH DONATIONS

A. Edgar Benton, Aerospace Physiologist Society, Alpine Club of Canada, American Chemical Society (Bakersfield), American College of Chest Physicians, ANCO Engineers, Attilio D. Renzetti, Jr., M.D., Ben Eiseman, M.D., Brown Canon, Jr., Charles and Luanne Hazelrigg, Charles B. Leonard, Charles J. Kall, David Dantzker, M.D., David Michels, Ph.D., David Shepro, Ph.D., Department of Physiology, University of Pennsylvania, Donald W. & Sandra Solmonson, Douglas G. McNair, Mrs. Eleonore Frank, Esther Hardenbergh, F. Charles and Stuie Froehlicher, Francis S. Belknap, Frank R. Isenhart, Fred J. Meyers, Gilbert Frye, Gordon M. Callison, Harry T. Lewis, Jr., Health Science Foundation, Henry Hall, Jr., Hermann Rahn, Ph.D., Hugh MacMillan, M.D., Hugh and Marty Downey, Jacob Kornwasser, James A. Richardson, John H. Batten, John B. Holyoke, Joseph C. Anderson, Joy R. Hilliard, J&S Rentals, Drs. J. W. & M. McKibben, Leo Roon, Linda Stuart III, Lucy B. Hibbert, Maria A. Warren, Marvin Sackner, M.D., Medina Foundation, Morgan and Julie Smith, M. J. Murdock Charitable Trust, Norman Holter, D.Sc., Patrick and Brenda Owen, Pepsico Foundation, Perry Hall, Pierre Dejours, M.D., Robert Donner, Jr., Robert F. Rahn, Robert H. Ramsay, Robert P. Eckhardt, Dr. & Mrs. Robert Schoene Memorial Fund, Robert L. Putnam Research Fund, Scientific Research Society (China Lake), Sidney Graber, Susan S. Writer, Ted and Kise LaMontagne, The Northcliff Fund, Thomas W. Swanson, Times Mirror, Twin Disc Inc., Ulrich Luft, M.D., United Bank of Denver, Verne Reed, V. Q. Telford, M.D., William Belknap, Jr., William C. Dabney, William Putnam, William S. Hershberger.

SPONSORS

The American Alpine Club, American Physiological Society, Explorers Club.

INDEX

187